Praise for Brilliance & Confusion

Brilliance & Confusion: Saving Children's Vision and Lives with Vitamin A is the best kind of science storytelling: rigorously true, consistently interesting, and filled with the excitement of discovery and unexpected insights into how the human body — and science itself — really works. Prof. Vern Paetkau, himself a renowned biochemist, traces the story of vitamin A from its earliest discovery to current efforts to make vitamin A deficiency a thing of the past. His engaging book leaves readers with a greater appreciation for "the micronutrient that bears the first letter of the vitamin alphabet," and for the many scientists who helped unlock the secrets of its nature and importance along the way.

— THOMAS HAYDEN, PROFESSOR OF THE PRACTICE, STANFORD UNIVERSITY SCHOOL OF EARTH, ENERGY & ENVIRONMENTAL SCIENCES

Brilliance & Confusion: Saving Children's Vision and Lives with Vitamin A is a wonderful read — indeed, a must-read for anyone interested in vitamins and other essential nutrients, the politics of science, and the misinterpretations, intentional or not, of clinical trials. It is exceptionally comprehensive. Starting with the influential and important studies of Alfred Sommer and his team on vitamin A deficiency in Indonesian children in the late 1970s, it then goes back to the early evidence that there are essential nutrients that must be in one's diet to survive, and the discovery of vitamin A at the beginning of the 20th century as one of those nutrients. It explains the role of vitamin A not only in vision, but for the maintenance of epithelial tissues and in preventing disease and death. The two critical derivatives of vitamin A are described — retinal (vitamin A aldehyde) for vision, and retinoic acid (vitamin A acid) for somatic functions. The book moves on to discuss treating vitamin A deficiency in humans, especially children, and its success in the West and many developing countries throughout the world, the exception being the rice-dependent Asian countries. A last chapter is devoted to the story of golden rice, which potentially could solve this problem. The resistance over the years to programs designed to eradicate the deficiency in various countries is presented, including the more recent attempts to prevent the development of golden rice. The discussion is not limited just to vitamin A but extends to other vitamins and micronutrients as well. Sprinkled with anecdotes and brief biographies of many of the major players over the years, the book is a pleasure to read, and I learned much from it. I recommend it highly.

— JOHN E. DOWLING, GORDON AND LLURA GUND RESEARCH PROFESSOR OF NEUROSCIENCES, HARVARD UNIVERSITY, PIONEER RESEARCHER OF VITAMIN A'S ROLE IN VISION AND ESSENTIAL CELLULAR FUNCTIONS, AND IN THE NEUROBIOLOGY OF VISION.

I have been a constant reader of the history of science since encountering *The Structure of Scientific Revolutions* in graduate school. There are many "popular" histories that fail to do justice to the complexities of the science. Other works by scientists are sometimes beyond the comprehension of non-specialists. This fascinating history of the double discovery of vitamin A and its multiple roles in human development does full justice to the science and is an engaging read. *Brilliance & Confusion: Saving Children's Vision and Lives with Vitamin A* not only has roots deep in the beginnings of biomedical science but addresses a vitally important policy issue in today's world.

— RODERICK C. MACLEOD, PROFESSOR EMERITUS OF HISTORY AND CLASSICS, UNIVERSITY OF ALBERTA. AUTHOR OF *PRAIRIE FIRE: THE 1885 NORTH WEST REBELLION AND ALL TRUE THINGS: A HISTORY OF THE UNIVERSITY OF ALBERTA, 1908–2008.*

BRILLIANCE & CONFUSION:
SAVING CHILDREN'S VISION & LIVES WITH VITAMIN A

VERN PAETKAU

Editing by Dania Sheldon

Book design by Alex Hennig

ISBN 978-0-9810523-1-1 (paperback)

ISBN 978-0-9810523-2-8 (eBook)

Published by Createspace

Brilliance and Confusion: Saving Children's Vision and Lives with Vitamin A

Contents

Introduction

This book is about vitamin A, an essential micronutrient for humans. It proposes to take you on an illuminating journey, beginning with an understanding of how we came to discover vitamins and their roles in nutrition. Vitamin A, the "vision vitamin," has an essential role in human well-being and life itself, a fact that was discovered and then rediscovered decades later. This understanding led to an investigation of the effects of vitamin A deficiency in the developing world, which threatens the vision, well-being, and very lives of millions of children. The book describes how this essential micronutrient can be provided in a sustainable way, ending with a detailed look at a controversial effort to use the power of genetic engineering to this end.

In Chapter 1, I relate the rediscovery in the 1980s of the life-essential properties of vitamin A, some 55 years after this had been previously documented but which had then been largely forgotten. The next chapter outlines the history of vitamin discovery more generally and explains how the realization that dietary deficiency can cause disease profoundly changed the way we view human health. In Chapter 3, I describe the structure and functions of the various forms of vitamin A and how the vitamin's two unrelated biological activities are responsible for maintaining vision, on the one hand, and life itself, on the other. Chapter 4 explains the effects of vitamin A on human health. Chapter 5 describes some strategies for overcoming vitamin A deficiency and also the limits on those strategies, which may not be feasible, or robust, for some segments of the world's population. Chapter 6 then presents and explores a controversial solution to the problem of vitamin A deficiency for the three billion people of the world who depend on rice for their well-being. Finally, I close with a consideration of future directions and advocate for an evidence-based, collaborative approach to globally eradicate the devastating effects of vitamin A deficiency.

CHAPTER 1

Vitamin A, Essential for Vision and Life

An epiphany in Baltimore

It was Christmas week of 1982, a quiet time away from clinical duties, research, and teaching, when Dr. Alfred Sommer, professor of ophthalmology at Johns Hopkins University, decided to take another look at the results of a large public health study he had been involved in. The fieldwork for that study had taken place between March 1977 and December 1978, in rural West Java, Indonesia. The government of that country wanted to understand the degree of vitamin A deficiency among children in rural areas and the associated risk factors. Vitamin A was known to be important for sight — one form of the vitamin is part of the visual pigment of the eye — and without enough vitamin A in the diet, a child will start to lose vision. Vitamin A deficiency results in a condition called xerophthalmia, a series of steps of deterioration of the eyes that begins with an inability to see in low light, or "nightblindness." If the vitamin deficiency continues, the damage becomes worse, leading ultimately to complete blindness and the destruction of eye tissue. The government of Indonesia wanted to know whether there were factors in the lives of children that made vitamin A deficiency, and the resulting problems with their vision, more likely. Many children in rural Indonesia suffered from nightblindness, although they often soon recovered. But carrying out a field study in those areas was challenging. It required a multifaceted team of investigators and careful assessment of the study's conditions and goals. In response to a request from the Indonesian government, Sommer had put together a team uniquely qualified to answer those questions.

Sommer had earned his medical degree at Harvard in 1967 and already had a hankering — which he shared with his wife — to serve in the Peace Corps. But Congress passed legislation the following year that essentially guaranteed he would be drafted out of the Peace Corps and sent to Vietnam. The fighting there was heavy, and doctors were badly needed. So instead, he enrolled with the Center for Disease Control, in Atlanta, Georgia. He found the pace at this government institution a bit slow, and when he became aware of a chance to go to East Pakistan to join a group trying to contain a cholera outbreak, he jumped at the opportunity. He served in East Pakistan from 1969 to 1972. This was his first experience living and working in a hot, uncomfortable, challenging, developing-world environment, and he loved it. It was a time of political upheaval, as East Pakistan was breaking away from its larger West Pakistan overlords to become Bangladesh, a development in which Sommer had a small but non-trivial part, as described in his entertaining account of that time (1).

At that point, Sommer had yet to undergo any specialist training, but what interested him was epidemiology, the study of disease patterns in populations, and ophthalmology, the treatment of eye diseases. This combination of specialties was, and remains, uncommon. Upon his return to the United States from Bangladesh, he undertook the necessary further training in those sub-disciplines while retaining a strong interest in working in developing countries. Sommer obtained a degree in epidemiology in 1973 and immediately enrolled in the residency program in ophthalmology at Johns Hopkins University. During this time, he met a woman named Susan Pettis, who was the Director of Blindness Prevention for the American Foundation for Overseas Blind, now known as Helen Keller International. Because of his experience in East Pakistan, Sommer was able to help that organization, and Pettis became something of a mentor to him. In 1974, Sommer had a chance to go to Indonesia with her to attend the first international conference to address blindness caused by nutritional deficiencies, "nutritional blindness," of which vitamin A deficiency is a prime example. The conference was organized by the World

Health Organization (WHO), and Sommer considered himself lucky to be able to attend, given his junior status.

Despite his youth, Sommer took an active part in the meeting proceedings. On the last day, he was sitting on one side of Susan Pettis, and a high-ranking official of the Indonesian Ministry of Health was sitting on the other. The government of Indonesia was interested in the problem of nutritional blindness and wanted to learn more about its epidemiology before starting a program of vitamin A capsule distribution to combat it. Sommer remarked to Pettis that Indonesia would be a wonderful country in which to investigate nutritional blindness. The Indonesian official overheard the remark and, as recalled by Sommer more than twenty years later, whispered to her, "Is there any way that we can get Dr. Sommer to come here for a few years and work with us?" Recalled Sommer further, "And she's sitting in the center and smiling to herself, and saying, 'I think I can make a deal here.'" As a result, Sommer found himself invited to start such a study, which he put off for a few years while he finished his residency in ophthalmology at Johns Hopkins.

In 1976, Sommer had completed his residency. His talents had been noticed, and his future looked bright, with a faculty appointment at Johns Hopkins a real possibility. He was given friendly advice that undertaking an epidemiological study in a far-off, developing country might harm his career — people back in the USA would forget him, and he could be damaging his chances of an academic medical position. Sommer disregarded that conventional wisdom and began to organize funding and people to look at the problem of vitamin A deficiency in Indonesia. With those in place, he gathered up his wife and two young children and left the United States for four years.

When the study in rural Indonesia began, it was already known that children there had a high rate of mild xerophthalmia, mainly characterized by nightblindness, but that most of the affected children spontaneously regained normal vision. The children being studied were from poor, rural backgrounds, and their high incidence of nightblindness was presumed to result from diets deficient in certain critical nutrients, particularly vitamin A. Fluctuations in the diet probably accounted for the transient nature of their nightblindness. One of the goals of the study was to see whether any other circumstances contributed to nightblindness.

The group put together by Sommer included a paediatrician, an ophthalmologist, a nutritionist, two nurses, and six local field workers. Close to 4,600 children were enrolled in the study. The presence of the field workers allowed the doctors to obtain extensive histories from their patients, including the mothers' recollections about their children's health. Blood samples were taken, and objective clinical tests for nightblindness were performed. Of those children with nightblindness, most got better spontaneously, as expected. Children showing signs of more serious eye damage due to progressive xerophthalmia were given vitamin A to help them recover.

The children were seen every three months over a period of a year and a half. The doctors often found themselves relying on the mothers' memories, as told to a local fieldworker — memories that almost always turned out to be correct, as seen by clinical examination. A mother might recall that her child had recently undergone a period of nightblindness, during which the child could not see at dusk or dawn, could not find their food, would huddle in a corner of the hut, and would not walk about in the village during periods of low light.

The doctors determined that the incidence of mild xerophthalmia increased until about age three. As predicted, children with xerophthalmia had low levels of vitamin A in their blood. Children whose diet was low in foods that provide vitamin A, such as dark green leafy vegetables and orange or yellow vegetables or fruits, were more likely to be vitamin A deficient. So were children with respiratory diseases or diarrhoea, which draw down vitamin A levels. And vitamin A deficiency was associated with nightblindness. All of this made sense and wasn't unexpected.

Sommer believed that after so much effort and expense, it was important to analyze the results of such studies intensively and repeatedly, to obtain every morsel of understanding the data could provide beyond the initial answers to the leading questions. That's what he was doing during Christmas week four years after the fieldwork had ended. As he repeatedly reviewed the data from the Indonesian study, something nagged at him.

In studies of this type, it's important to retain the study subjects; if too many drop out, the results may be biased and conclusions can be compromised. A point of pride in this particular study was that by diligent effort, most of the children enrolled could be followed to the end of it. But retention is never 100%; some people move away, or sometimes they are busy working in the fields when it comes time for the next visit to the clinic. So, there was a decrease in the number of children seen as the study progressed. This was expected. But what suddenly caught Sommer's attention was that these losses were disproportionately from the group of children who at one point or another had experienced nightblindness or other symptoms of early, mild xerophthalmia. Why? An examination of additional data provided the answer: they had died. Children with the very mildest, early stages of xerophthalmia, nightblindness, were dying at three times the rate of those not showing such symptoms, even though they usually recovered their vision. Children with a more severe condition, with more progressive xerophthalmia, died at six times the rate of healthy children. Children with advanced xerophthalmia, but still not near total blindness, died at nine times the rate of children with no symptoms. Not only were the children losing their vision, they were losing their lives. Mild xerophthalmia, a condition that usually reverses spontaneously, was associated with an increased risk of death. At the time, this was completely unexpected.

Scientists really do have revelatory experiences, although they don't usually shout, "Eureka!" That moment when a scientist realizes that he or she has seen something that nobody else has seen, when the understanding of a scientific story changes, even to a small degree, is golden and often shapes the rest of his or her life. A single observation cannot establish the validity of a dramatic new result — it requires corroboration — but the path by which the new finding can be tested and either accepted or rejected is now clear.[1] A flash of insight has illuminated something that had not been seen previously, and interrogating the natural world to determine

---

1 Further testing of a new finding to prove its veracity is of course required, but at some point in a working scientist's life there may be an event that carries an aura of inevitability about it at its first observation. Or at least, that's how we remember it.

whether that insight reflects reality is what scientists are trained to do. Alfred Sommer thought he was seeing something new and important, linking mild xerophthalmia, a condition thought to be benign and easily reversible, to an increased risk of death. In interviews, he refers to this revelation as his "holy cow" moment, although in his memoir of the time he admits that "cow" wasn't actually the word he used (1).

The initial study by Sommer and his colleagues was an observational investigation that suggested a link between vitamin A deficiency, mild xerophthalmia, and childhood death. A logical conclusion would have been that vitamin A deficiency causes nightblindness, which in turn can lead to death. But correlation isn't proof of causality. The critical next step would have to be a study that specifically asked: Does vitamin A supplementation in a large group of nutritionally challenged children prevent nightblindness and early childhood death? At the moment of Sommer's epiphany, he was busy setting up another, larger study in Indonesia, which would extend the findings of the first one. By modifying this study, the researchers could directly test the hypothesis that vitamin A supplementation prevents childhood deaths. Over the next years, the work of the Johns Hopkins team and others confirmed Sommer's initial suspicion, but reaction to and repercussions from those studies still engage medical science and health policy today. Discoveries about the importance of vitamin A in the diet have led to beneficial intervention on a global scale by non-governmental agencies. But there have also been ideological and nationalistic reactions to those interventions. The issue of vitamin A deficiency has taken medical science to the leading edge of biological research, through the creation of genetically engineered crops that may be an answer to vitamin A deficiency. There also has been profound opposition to that approach.

At the heart of these issues is the health of millions of children in the developing world. For as the first observational study suggested, their very lives, as well as their vision, depend on their ability to obtain the micronutrient that bears the first letter of the vitamin alphabet. It is a micronutrient essential for life. This book is the story of how that vitamin was identified during a golden age of vitamin discovery, what it does in the human body, how it affects our health, and how it presently is — and in the future can be — provided to those who do not currently get enough of it.

What is vitamin A?

"Vitamin A" is a generic term for a small group of related, fat-soluble compounds. Retinol and two closely related chemical forms called retinal and retinoic acid constitute the vitamin A found in animals' bodies, where they carry out a number of essential functions. They are referred to as "preformed" vitamin A, whose structures and functions will be described in detail in Chapter 3. Retinol is stored in animals' livers and is present in dairy products, eggs, and a number of other animal-derived foods.

Vitamin A is also present in many food plants in "provitamin" forms called carotenoids. That name suggests carrots, and in fact, carrots are a good source of these provitamins, as are some other yellow or orange vegetables, such as sweet potatoes, as well as dark green leafy vegetables, such as spinach. Beta-carotene, the most common provitamin A, is split by cells in the human gut into two molecules of functional vitamin A; these are absorbed into the blood and either used immediately or stored in the liver for later use. Only animal tissues contain "preformed" vitamin A. Plants contain only provitamin A forms such as beta-carotene and other carotenoids.

People have been indirectly aware of the existence of vitamin A for thousands of years, well before we knew what it is. Today, those of us fortunate enough to enjoy a balanced and nutritious diet don't need to be concerned about vitamin A deficiency; it's present in many of our foods, including whole milk (and skim milk, to which it is added after the fat has been skimmed off), other dairy-based foods, eggs, meats, and several kinds of vegetables. But in parts of the world where diets are not well rounded, such as large areas of sub-Saharan Africa, India, Asia, and parts of Central America, vitamin A deficiency threatens the health and the lives of millions, particularly children. The results of the early studies of Sommer and his colleagues reflected that threat. The WHO concluded in 2009 that between 190 and 250 million people worldwide, including 19 million pregnant women, are vitamin A deficient (2). Estimates of the number of children globally whose very lives are at risk run to the hundreds of thousands *a year*.[2] To have such numbers of people at risk is unacceptable, especially as solutions for the problem exist. The question is, which solutions are effective, sustainable, and acceptable?

Just over a hundred years ago, nutritional scientists in the United States showed that there was a fat-soluble, trace nutrient in animal liver, dairy products, the dark green leaves of many plants, and a number of yellow or orange foods that was necessary for health and for life itself. They gave it the name "fat-soluble A" because it was the first identified fat-soluble essential trace nutrient. Within a few years, its name was changed to "vitamin A." The term "vitamin" was a revision of "vital amines," the first general descriptor for the vitamins as a class of micronutrients. Over time, several other fat-soluble vitamins were discovered. The water-soluble vitamins, several of whose essential roles in nutrition had been identified even before "fat-soluble A," were mostly grouped as "B vitamins." The B vitamins were later separated into seven different chemical entities, whose individual functions cover a wide spectrum of essential metabolic activities. Another water-soluble vitamin, C, was one of the earliest essential micronutrients to have its effects identified.

We live in a time of high demand for dietary news. As coverage has grown ever more extensive in the area of lifestyle and the many food-related issues that surround us, interrogating Google for articles on "nutrition" will apparently produce 419 million articles in 0.34 seconds. This number includes articles in sources that we wouldn't expect to have much interest in dietary news, and they range from the commonsensical (*The New Republic*: "Many doctors dismiss nutritional therapies as quack medicine. But many patients disagree, and they're taking matters into their own hands — sometimes to the detriment of their health."), to the satisfying (*The Economist*: "Chocolate is blamed for causing cavities and making people fat, but in modest quantities it is actually a healthy treat."), to the

---

2 For reasons that I will explore later, it is difficult to know how many children die each year of vitamin A deficiency. The WHO estimates 125,000; most other estimates are higher.

unsubstantiated ("Dr. Oz's Three-Day Detox Cleanse"). Other than enriching a few entrepreneurs, almost none of this "news" will have much of an effect on anyone, beyond perhaps a brief period of weight loss or of anecdotal well-being, or ill health, almost always followed by a return to a previous state of mind and body. But there is a large, important nutrition-related story just beyond our everyday experience, and it is one seldom commented on. It concerns the profound health effects of vitamin A deficiency. That deficiency can be quantitatively demonstrated — blood levels of vitamin A in those affected are low to non-existent, they have insufficient vitamin A stored in their livers, and they suffer exactly the symptoms of incipient blindness, failure to thrive, and consequent death that have been known to accompany vitamin A deficiency in studies on animals and clinical trials in humans.

There are multiple reasons why the problems of vitamin A deficiency are not generally better known in the developed world and why effective solutions have not been developed. In the first place, we tend to see it as a "third-world" problem, well removed from most first-world eyes. It's a depressing and apparently unsolvable problem from a Western point of view — poor or insufficient nutrition is still widespread, and despite progress in increasing the quantity of food produced in the developing world, we have yet to adequately solve issues of nutritional quality. Vitamin A deficiency is directly connected to poverty, and even when solutions exist, those affected often can't afford them and depend on donors, who may grow fatigued in their efforts. Progress in solving the problem has been slow, and sometimes it stalls for irrational reasons. Against all of this, it is clearly the case that solutions already exist, that newer solutions are available for testing, and that none of these solutions costs very much on a global scale. There are people with a strong concept of how to overcome the damaging effects of vitamin A deficiency, but the enabling plans are sometimes blocked by interfering priorities and interests, as I will describe.

Vitamin deficiencies have been known, by various names, for thousands of years. Nightblindness due to vitamin A deficiency was apparent to ancient Egyptians, as was its solution — eating ox liver (which works). Vitamin C deficiency was an impediment to Britain's efforts at global domination through its naval might; sailors were dying, suddenly and inexplicably, when they spent more than a few weeks away from land. And as peasant farmers moved from the land to jobs in smoke-beclouded cities during the industrial revolution, their children began to suffer from the crippling effects of vitamin D deficiency due to a lack of solar ultraviolet light. Their bones were ill-formed, and their lives often ended prematurely.

The problem of scurvy, caused by a lack of vitamin C, was solved in the early nineteenth century, but most vitamin discovery began only toward the end of that century. At that time, even as research indicated that certain trace nutrients are essential for health and for life itself, the hypothesis that a deficiency in a trace nutrient could cause disease was denigrated by many scientists and doctors, who were wedded to two valid but incomplete paradigms: that diseases are caused by infectious microorganisms (many are, but some very important ones, like cancer, heart disease, and vitamin deficiencies, usually are not), and that what matters in nutrition is quantity — eat enough food and you will be healthy. The latter idea derived from the metaphor that your body is an engine, and you need to provide it with enough fuel or it will fail. But gradually, increasing levels of scientific rigour, which demanded that claims be backed up by verifiable, reproducible evidence, led thoughtful people to the ineluctable conclusion that some micronutrients are indeed essential for animal, including human, well-being, and that deficiencies in these can cause dangerous illness and even death. Eventually, humans were found to need 13 vitamins in all, one after another of which was identified between about 1880 and 1945. The structure of each was determined in due course, and its role in human biology was mapped.

As this classical phase of vitamin discovery was winding down, it was assumed that we understood almost everything we needed to know about the vitamins. Like Lord Kelvin's pronouncement in 1900 that there was nothing new to be discovered in physics, the notion that our understanding of vitamins was now complete was not correct, even in 1945. And nowhere did that inadequacy become more evident than in the biology of vitamin A, the most complex of all the vitamins in its actions and activities. In retrospect, we should have recognized its significant and complex effects on human health because of research in the 1920s and 1930s. But we failed to grasp the full meaning of that work, until suddenly the evidence that vitamin A deficiency was the key element in a large global health problem was overwhelming.

The late Arthur Kornberg, discoverer of the enzyme system that duplicates genomic DNA, described himself and many of the biological scientists of the 1940s and 1950s as "enzyme hunters." Enzymes are the biological catalysts that carry out all of the chemical reactions in living cells, from breaking down sugar for energy to expressing genes, and the search for these proteins was particularly intense during that time, although it had begun earlier and continues today. Kornberg described the progress of biomedical research as a succession of periods. The "microbe hunters" described by the popular science writer Paul de Kruif occupied the spotlight in the first two decades of the 20th century, as they discovered one microbe after another responsible for human diseases. The next 20 years featured the "vitamin hunters," followed by the "enzyme hunters" and then the "gene hunters." Kornberg noted that each age, "with its particularly bountiful quarry, was seen as golden" (3). Be that as it may, the early decades of the 20th century did indeed see tremendous progress in the discovery of various organic trace nutrients, or micronutrients, that came to be identified as the vitamins essential for our well-being. The hunt for vitamins was facilitated by the fact that laboratory animals also need most of the same vitamins as humans do and hence can be used to identify and characterize them.

This is more than a story about a branch of human nutrition; there are serious current issues of life and death related to vitamin A that go well beyond the science and medicine. To properly deal with these issues requires a cool-headed and logical approach, together with a will to help those who cannot help themselves. There are contentious issues and competing visions in play when we consider what is to be done. What makes the matter especially urgent is that very young children are most at risk. The obvious risk is to their eyesight, but as the experience of Sommer and his research team indicated, there is a profound risk to their broader well-being and their very lives. The effects of vitamin A on their health are a reflection of the biological roles of this most complex of the vitamins. Its name reflects that it was one of the first to be discovered, but its complexities continue to be revealed to this day.

CHAPTER 2

Vitamin Discovery: A Time of Brilliance and Confusion

Calories are not enough

When Dr. Maurice Gueniot, an important member of the French medical establishment, died in 1935, he had an impressive record of achievements, including the presidency of the Paris Medical Academy. In addition to his establishment credentials, he was widely known as a practicing disciple of a faith that believed, with almost no evidence, that chronic undernourishment, eating less than you wanted to, could extend lifespan. The theory behind this belief was that if the human "engine" consumed less fuel, it might wear out more slowly. To follow his dietary principle, the incredibly disciplined Dr. Gueniot limited his food intake to more or less starvation rations for most of his adult life. While a sample size of one (him) doesn't give his experimental result any statistical weight, he did live for 102 years. It probably seemed even longer; more recent practitioners of calorie restriction often report an unrelenting hunger.[3]

The year 1935 saw another important contribution to the longevity–undernourishment theory, and the follow-up work from that study still engages both biomedical scientists and lay people interested in extending lifespan. This study carried more statistical weight and scientific credibility than Gueniot's solo effort. It was about rats, not humans, but by

---

3   There are surprisingly many people today who are trying to extend their lifespan by restricting calories. The jury is still out on whether the approach works for humans. Perhaps it's significant that on the Japanese island of Okinawa, where life expectancy is higher than almost anywhere else on earth, people are said to stop eating before experiencing satiety; "80% satiated" is the term used. For rats, the issue appears to be settled, as McCay and Crowell's 1935 study demonstrated.

then, rats had been accepted as a reasonable substitute for many aspects of human nutrition. The work was directed by Drs. Clive McCay and Mary Crowell at Cornell University, in Ithaca, New York. McCay had been intrigued by another story of food self-denial, of older origin. A 40-year-old Italian diabetic living in the 16th century, a man who seemed to be dying, put himself on a strict calorie-reduced diet. Within a week, he claimed to feel better, and he lived an apparently full and hearty life of 98 years. McCay was intrigued; was calorie restriction a gateway to longer life? To try to answer this question, McCay set up an experiment on rats, in which he fed some of them normal rations and restricted the others to just 60% of their usual intake.

The results were astonishing (4). Normally, when rats are fed ad lib (eating as much as they want), male rats grow to a larger size than females but usually die younger. But when, by limiting their intake of calories, the growth rate of male rats was slowed down and even stopped for a period of their lives, they lived longer, in some cases even longer than the average female rat. Of the male rats fed ad lib, half died by day 500, which was the usual lifespan for these animals. But for the calorie-restricted male rats, the comparable period was over 800 days. (The female rats, smaller than their male littermates, lived for an average of 800 days even on an ad lib diet. Their lifespan was less affected by calorie restriction.)

Other scientists before McCay and Crowell had tried to do the same kind of experiment. Most of them were approaching the subject from the opposite direction — the animal body needed fuel, and starving it would lead to its failure. They expected lifespan to be shorter for calorie-restricted animals. Their expectations were based on new directions in nutrition research. Toward the end of the 19th century, it had turned to the harder sciences for new insights. Scientists incorporated the laws of thermodynamics into their understanding of nutrition and realized that living bodies were at least a little like engines or furnaces. They needed fuel, and the energy value of that fuel could be quantitatively measured; this principle is what's behind our assignment of caloric content to different foods. Moreover, the ability of a living body, whether human or rat, to do work was limited by its fuel intake. Energy could be provided interchangeably by different kinds of food; calories obtained from carbohydrate, protein, and fat were more or less interchangeable. What mainly mattered in the new view was the total energy taken in. The primary consideration was to provide enough energy content in the diet. A prominent source of advice to women about motherhood and nutrition during the early decades of the 20th century was the American Anna Steese Richardson. She advised: "Stoke the engine of your body with the right sort of coal, keep it clear of cinders and clinkers, cleanse it with pure water, renew the worn parts with rest. . . . What is the right kind of coal? Food-stuffs classified according to their chemical properties . . . water, mineral matter, proteins, carbohydrates, and fats" (quoted in (5)) — a philosophy precisely opposite to Dr. Gueniot's.

Given the prevailing view that food was simply fuel, it isn't surprising that some scientists thought undernourishment would be harmful, so calorie restriction might reduce lifespan. But when scientists tested this hypothesis on laboratory animals, the experimental results were all over the map; in some cases, scientists did see a decrease in longevity following starvation, but in others, there was no change, or even an increase. The variability of their results arose from an important design flaw in their calorie-restricted experimental diets. The subjects were missing more than just calories; in many instances, the animals were also being starved of trace nutrients. McCay's understanding was more sophisticated; he knew about the importance of trace nutrients, including salts such as calcium, magnesium, and iron, and also of a group of micronutrients that had begun to be defined and described over the previous decades — the vitamins. McCay and Crowell enriched their experimental diets so that all rats received adequate quantities of the precious trace nutrients despite any calorie restriction, and they got the clear and reproducible result that had eluded other scientists, for whom the insufficiency of micronutrients (which reduced lifespan) worked against calorie reduction (which increased it).

The failure of scientists before McCay and Crowell to get consistent, reliable results in their calorie-restriction experiments reflected the fact that nutrition was poorly understood in the early 20th century. The focus was on the energy content of various kinds of food, founded upon the belief that what mattered was mainly having *enough* to eat; having access to each of the major food groups — fat, protein, and carbohydrate — was probably also important. But some studies even before 1900 were casting uncertainty on this limited view, and it was gradually becoming clear that something was missing in the simple calorie-counting approach. That "something," as McCay and Crowell recognized, involved trace nutrients, or micronutrients, including salts and vitamins.

The first scientific evidence for a new type of essential nutrient

The "golden age" of vitamin discovery started with a group of doctors and scientists living in the Netherlands toward the end of the 19th century. One of these was Christiaan Eijkman, who was born in Nijkierk, Gelderland, the Netherlands, on August 11, 1858. He was the seventh child of Christiaan, a school headmaster, and Johanna, a housewife. There was not much in the way of family history to suggest that the younger Christiaan would become known first as an esteemed physician specializing in tropical diseases, then as the discoverer of the water-soluble vitamin we call thiamin. That discovery foreshadowed other research on the effects of vitamins on nutrition and health and won him a Nobel Prize.

Eijkman enrolled in the Military Medical School of the University of Amsterdam, where he qualified as a medical officer of the Royal Netherlands East Indies Army. After completing his doctorate in 1883, he sailed for the Dutch East Indies, today's Indonesia, to look after the health of its colonial masters and the native workers who toiled to produce the wealth that sustained the Dutch empire. But just two years later he caught malaria and had to return to Europe. There he began work under senior scientists to develop his research capabilities. A while later he found himself in the laboratory of Robert Koch in Berlin. At the time, Koch was the world's most highly regarded expert in infectious diseases, and his name is still revered for his contributions to that field.

While Eijkman was working in Koch's laboratory, two other Dutch scientists arrived there, one of whom was Cornelius Pekelharing.

Pekelharing and his colleague, Dr. Winkler, an expert in neurology, were being sent to the Dutch East Indies to study a deadly and baffling neurological disease called beriberi.[4] The symptoms included paralysis, numbness and weakness of the limbs, and cardiac and respiratory failure, and the disease could strike down a strong man almost in his tracks. A soldier might be in good health in the morning, able to show off his prowess at target practice, and fall victim to the disease by evening. Victims characteristically experienced difficulty in walking. Beriberi particularly afflicted groups of men living "under constraint," such as soldiers, sailors, prisoners, and indentured Javanese workers.

Beriberi was thought to be an infectious disease, which was why Pekelharing and Winkler had come to Berlin to find out about the latest techniques of bacteriology from the master, Koch. By the time they set off for the Dutch East Indies, Eijkman, having recovered from malaria and being willing to subject himself to tropical conditions again, had committed to joining them as soon as he could. The purpose of the expedition was to identify the bacteria that caused beriberi; instead, it became the start of the science of vitamins in nutrition.

Early results by the Pekelharing team were consistent with the idea that there was an infectious agent in the blood of beriberi patients that could sometimes cause neural degeneration in test animals. He recommended a vigorous campaign of sterilization and cleanliness, and the incidence of beriberi among the native workers did decline for a while, but then it increased again. Frustrated, but having to return to his position at the University of Utrecht, Pekelharing recommended that the research institute in Batavia (today's Jakarta, the capital of Indonesia) be made permanent, with Eijkman, who had joined the team by then, as its first director. Pekelharing went on to make other important discoveries in medicine, but his work was mostly published in Dutch, and for many years it remained out of the view of scientists not familiar with that language. (This was a recurring problem before the ascent of English as the *lingua franca* of science.) Eijkman, in turn, went on to win the Nobel Prize in

---

4 The name beriberi may have originated in the Sinhalese language in Ceylon (now Sri Lanka), in which it means "I can't, I can't," apparently in reference to the muscular weakness of those afflicted.

Physiology or Medicine for discovering the basis of beriberi, which was not an infectious disease at all but a nutritional one.

When Eijkman began working in Java, almost nobody gave any credence to the idea that something missing from the diet might cause illness — the germ theory of disease was dominant. In the mid-19th century, Louis Pasteur had demonstrated that fermentation and spoilage were due to living organisms, and that spontaneous generation of life (a theory proposing that piles of dirty rags, for example, could generate living organisms) was nonsense. To produce living organisms, Pasteur showed, you needed to start with living organisms. He further proposed that diseases were caused by microorganisms. His work stimulated Joseph Lister to develop sterile methods of surgery, one of two advances that gave birth to modern surgery (the other being the invention of anaesthetics). Koch and other scientists had firmly established that "germs," bacteria, were important in a wide range of human diseases, and infection became the default theory for the cause of diseases, as reflected in Pekelharing's ideas about beriberi. The clustering of beriberi in certain localities, its periodic waxing and waning in different tropical countries, and other characteristics all inclined thinking toward the idea that it was an infectious disease.

After Pekelharing returned to the Netherlands, Eijkman and the rest of the Dutch team continued to study beriberi, but they had no success in identifying either an infectious agent or any other cause for the disease. Pekelharing's meagre results when trying to infect animals with blood from beriberi patients were not reproducible. The study of beriberi was at an impasse.

Then the chickens began to die — in particular, the chickens that were being kept to feed the laboratory staff of Eijkman's institute. The chickens were getting many of the same symptoms as humans with beriberi; their legs became feeble, and they began to walk oddly, often falling over in mid-stride. The afflicted chickens became too weak to get up or to eat, their breathing slowed, and they died. It seemed clear to the Dutch doctors that the chickens had a form of beriberi, and neurological examination confirmed it. There was no evidence for an infectious agent — the disease could not be transmitted from affected birds to healthy ones.

And then, just as suddenly as they had become afflicted, the chickens stopped getting sick and dying. Eijkman asked some questions and made observations, and soon realized that the health of the chickens waned and waxed with the identity of the staff person in charge of feeding them. For a time, they had been fed leftover cooked rice from the kitchen. As was customary, it was white rice, polished using Dutch equipment to remove the bran, since this gave it a longer shelf life under tropical conditions (the bran contains fats, which become rancid). Then the original chicken wrangler left and a new man was given the job. The new man was not about to feed the chickens "military rice" (the station was under the wing of the colonial Dutch military); they would eat "cruder," unpolished, brown rice. The chickens that were still alive immediately got better, and no more got sick. It was a clue. The source of the problem was identified when rice bran was found to cure beriberi. Interestingly, so did an extract of yeast. Evidently, poor nutrition could cause disease.

Eijkman saw an opportunity to test the theory's applicability to humans. It relied on observations of prisoners in the East Indies (fortunately for the study, there were many). This study, under Eijkman's direction, found that in prisons where the inmates ate polished rice there was a significant incidence of beriberi, while in those where brown rice was consumed, there wasn't. By this time, Eijkman was back in the Netherlands as a professor at the University of Utrecht, where he occupied himself with various other lines of medical research. But the observations he had made in Java were a breakthrough to an understanding of the water-soluble vitamins, which decades later led to the isolation and characterization of the first of these, the anti-neuritic agent vitamin B1, thiamin.

In Eijkman's 1929 Nobel Prize address, which he was not present to deliver, he had some comments to make about the cultural basis of the deficiency disease he had identified (6). He pointed out that before Dutch occupation, people in the countryside grew their own rice and shelled it by primitive means. This rice still contained the bran and thus provided thiamin. He commented ironically that "polished rice is processed mechanically and is one of the blessings of European civilization, of our improved techniques which, for instance, have also changed the colour of bread here in Europe from brown to white. . . . [T]he free population, which fed itself, was much less subject to beriberi than the population whose freedom was restricted, and which was often dependent on import- ed, and therefore mechanically processed, polished, rice."

Curiously, Eijkman was reluctant to accept the consensus explana- tion for why polished rice led to beriberi. He maintained, possibly right up to the time of his death in 1930, that the bran layer of the rice con- tained something that neutralised an unidentified toxic component of the rice germ. This was inconsistent with mounting evidence that it was a positive effect, not a toxin-neutralizing one, that accounted for the bene- ficial effects of the bran layer of rice. Gerrit Grijns, the doctor who took over in the Dutch East Indies when Eijkman returned to the Netherlands, showed clearly that other kinds of non-starch food, in particular boiled meat, could also cause beriberi in chickens, and that the condition could be reversed by extracts of rice bran or of yeast.

The official explanation for Eijkman not showing up to accept his Nobel Prize was that he was ill, which was true. But it may not have been the only, or even the main, reason; he may also have been disgruntled about how his work had been interpreted, and that others whose work was derivative of his were being honoured. His Nobel address contains a hint that he still thought that the vitamin in rice bran neutralized a neuritis-inducing material in the rice kernel. But even if he did believe this mistaken notion, his contributions had pushed an important line of research forward, and for this he is rightly honoured.

A complete diet needs more than just protein, fats, and carbohydrates

Eijkman's work took place in the last decades of the 19th century, but it did not immediately influence many of the conventional ideas about nutrition. Mainstream thinking said that the energy yield of food was what mattered, the calories it could provide. It was recognized that al- though carbohydrate, protein, and fat could substitute for each other in providing the necessary calories, at least some contribution by all three was necessary. The idea that there are essential micronutrients, trace components of the diet, didn't really take root before 1900. The first clear statement about essential organic micronutrients was made in a talk by the British biochemist Frederick Gowland Hopkins in 1906, which he later recalled in a 1912 paper (7): *"no animal can live upon a mixture of pure protein, fat, and carbohydrate. . . . The animal body is adjusted to live either upon plant tissues or the tissues of other animals, and these contain substances other than the proteins, carbohydrates, and fats."*

At the time he made this bold proclamation, Hopkins had only preliminary data to support it. He talked further about this idea in a lecture in 1909 but then fell ill and couldn't immediately carry out the necessary experiments. It took him until 1912 to test the hypothesis that more than just protein, fat, and carbohydrate (plus some salts) were required for life (7). He did this by creating an artificial diet consisting of the purified milk protein casein, which provides a good balance of the amino acids when digested, plus commercial starch and cane sugar, together with the salts present in milk. To reconstitute the fat component of the diet, he added lard, animal fat. Rats fed this synthetic diet grew for a while, but then they began to languish and die. This demonstrated that the reconstituted diet, although it contained an adequate supply of energy, a good source of protein, the required salts, and a copious source of carbohydrate, was inadequate in some way. Then came the critical next step: if to this synthetic diet Hopkins added a little whole milk, 1–4% by volume, the rats grew and remained healthy (see Figure 1). Clearly, milk contained a necessary micronutrient, one that was not present in the artificial diet and was essential for the rats to survive and thrive.

Hopkins then added weight to his interpretation of the results: When he switched the types of diets (artificial or milk-supplemented) between the two groups at day 18, at a time when the milk-less rats were beginning to go downhill, they soon began to gain weight and thrive, while the littermates that originally had been doing well began to lag behind and eventually wasted away. This showed that the milk-deprived animals hadn't been irreversibly poisoned in some way — at least at day 18 they could still be saved with the right dietary component from milk. It also showed that rats needed the essential milk micronutrient(s) on a continuing basis, and that removing this supplement led to decline and death. These are characteristic properties of the micronutrient we call vitamin A.

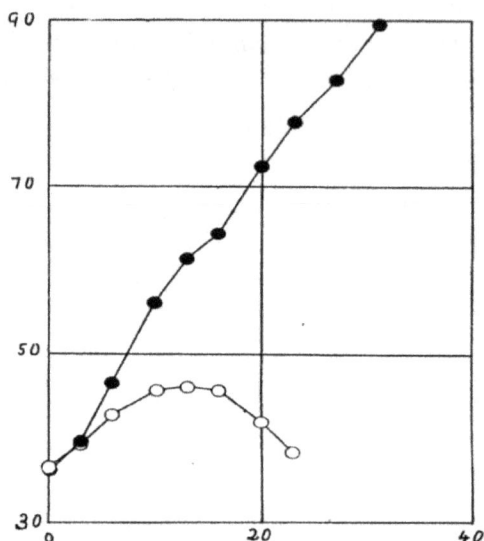

Fig. 1. Lower curve six rats on artificial diet alone. Upper curve six similar animals receiving in addition 2 c.c. of milk each per diem. Abscissæ time in days; ordinates average weight in grms.

Figure 1. The critical result from Hopkins' 1912 paper, showing that milk contained a nutrient essential for the growth and survival of rats. The vertical axis indicates the average weight of groups of six young rats over time, in grams. The horizontal axis indicates the time, in days. The open circles show the results for rats fed only the artificial diet. The solid circles show the results for rats given, in addition, 2 mL of milk each day. (From (7), with permission.)

Although Hopkins studied rats, it wasn't a stretch to think that the results might also apply to humans. His results were in a line of discovery that, unknown to him, began hundreds of years ago and extends to the present day, identifying vitamin A as necessary to sustain life. This is the crux of the story of this vitamin as it relates to human health.

In the picture of Hopkins on the website of the Nobel Prize organization, he has a serious, patrician air. He looks like someone who belongs to the aristocracy, and as far as science is concerned, he does, but he was anything but a snob. He was revered for his encouragement of and helpfulness to younger scientists, examples of which will emerge in this story. He was widely known as "Hoppy." This nature was consistent with his origins. He was born in humble middle-class circumstances. His father was a London bookseller who died when Frederick was an infant. The boy moved to the country with his mother and followed a fairly unremarkable path in his early education. Literature interested him, and he thought he might become a scholar of the classics, or perhaps a naturalist. But his academic strengths in science began to surface at age 10. He entered university to study chemistry in his 20s and became a forensic chemist. Among his tasks was establishing whether poisons had been used in committing certain infamous murders. At age 28 he entered medical school, and he became a physician at the relatively mature age of 32 (life expectancy the year he was born was about 45). A couple of years later he began to show his abilities as a scientist, combining his knowledge of medicine with his earlier expertise in chemistry. At 41, he was named the Professor of the newly created discipline of Biochemistry at Cambridge University, and the research contributions for which he would win a Nobel Prize began to appear.

When in 1929 he reviewed the work that led to his idea about organic micronutrients (the vitamins), Hopkins acknowledged that neither he nor anyone else had "invented" vitamins, and that even his nutritional studies showing that milk contained fat-soluble vitamins necessary for life were to some extent a repetition of earlier studies that he had been unaware of at the time. That was the work of a group in Basel, Switzerland, which had begun decades earlier. This group was headed by a German named Gustav von Bunge, who had achieved considerable fame by demonstrating that the growth of laboratory animals was limited by the number of calories they consumed. His results showed that it didn't much matter from which type of food those calories were derived, whether carbohydrate, fat, or protein. That work was consistent with the theory that its energy content was the limiting factor of a diet. However, a student in his laboratory, Nicolai Lunin, found that mice couldn't survive on a diet that contained only solvent-treated fats (a process that removes the fat-soluble vitamins), carbohydrates, proteins, and salts, but that a small amount of added whole milk would save them. He discovered this in 1881, some 30 years before Hopkins published essentially the same conclusion. Ten years later, another of von Bunge's students, C. A. Socin, found that egg yolk contained a component that could substitute for the critical constituent in milk. Again, this is a known property of vitamin A.

At the time he published his work on the importance of a fat-soluble micronutrient in the diet, in 1912, Hopkins was obviously reading (and quoting) the same German scientific publication (*Zeitschrift für Physiologische Chemie*) in which von Bunge's group had published their results in 1881 and 1891, but he apparently either had not read their earlier work or had not understood its full significance. While von Bunge and his students concluded that a natural food such as milk must contain small quantities of unknown substances that are essential to life, and had further determined that the missing nutrients could be found in other foods, von Bunge wasn't really convinced about the importance of organic micronutrients, and it wasn't surprising that others didn't rush to discover and study them as a result of his work. His own research group never followed up their initial hunch about non-mineral micronutrients, deciding instead to focus on the inorganic constituents of food — minerals such as calcium, iron, and magnesium. Even their paper that contained the quotation about essential substances was titled (translated from German) "The Importance of Inorganic Salts in Animal Nutrition." The work was never translated into English, and very few other scientists were aware of it.

Hopkins was also unaware of the work of the Dutch scientist Pekelharing, who, as we saw earlier, helped initiate the discovery of the B vitamin thiamin. Pekelharing had discovered the beneficial effects of milk on purified diets and published this result in 1905, in Dutch. However, communication of results across language barriers was neither easy nor common before the 20th century.

As for von Bunge, he was clearly an observant scientist, and his experience led him to several conclusions about diet that were well ahead of his time. He concluded, more than 160 years ago, that whole-grain bread was nutritionally better than white bread, that women receiving too little calcium in their diets had trouble breastfeeding, and that most people ate too much salt. He also thought that alcoholism was one of the most important reasons for human poverty and disease, and that smoking was partly responsible for many diseases of later life. Had he focused on the organic micronutrients essential to life, the vitamins, he might now be known as the father of vitamin research.

The birth of "fat-soluble A"

While communication between Hopkins and his Dutch and German colleagues was problematic, there was no barrier in his interactions with two groups working along similar lines in the United States. One of these was at the Connecticut Agricultural Experiment Station in New Haven, the other at the Laboratory of Agricultural Chemistry at the University of Wisconsin in Madison. The Connecticut group was led by Thomas Osborne and Lafayette Mendel, the one in Wisconsin by Elmer V. McCollum. The two American groups were familiar with each other — McCollum had worked with Osborne and Mendel when he was a student at Yale, and Mendel helped him secure a faculty position in Madison. Although the Americans were in contact with Hopkins by mail, they apparently had an incomplete understanding of what Hopkins had achieved. As a result, Hopkins was astonished to see, in 1913, a paper from Osborne and Mendel that claimed that no organic "growth hormones" (micronutrients) were required in the diet (they published that paper in *Zeitschrift für Physiologische Chemie*, which Hopkins was by now reading). Hopkins wrote them a letter complaining that "I have done so much work in this (very successful) endeavour to separate the unknown substances which affect growth, that when your paper . . . came out I suffered from an attack of nerves! . . . Casimir Funk brought me a copy . . . we were both somewhat overcome." (Funk was another contributor to early studies of vitamins.) Hopkins was upset that the American scientists hadn't appreciated his demonstration of the importance of a trace nutrient in milk. But thanks to the slow speed of communication, by the time he became aware of their 1913 publication in *Zeitschrift*, Osborne and Mendel had already switched to his view that trace organic nutrients *were* important, and they were working at top speed to identify them.

On June 1, 1913, a year after the publication of Hopkins' paper on the significance of small amounts of milk for rat nutrition, E. V. Mc-Collum and his research assistant Marguerite Davis published their own experiments on trace nutrients in milk. They used a similar synthetic diet to Hopkins', including lard as the source of fat, and their rats grew poorly, although not as poorly as Hopkins' rats; the difference was probably due to differences between their rat colonies, and how much vitamin A they had stored in their livers at the beginning of the experiments.[5] Then McCollum and Davis fed their languishing animals the fat-soluble components of those foods. Growth restarted immediately, and they concluded that some kind of organic, fat-soluble component was essential to the animals' diets (8). They acknowledged that it was similar in effect to the material present in the raw milk used by Hopkins (7), but they had taken the story a step forward by showing that whatever agent was responsible for resumed growth, it was fat-like (because it was extracted by ether), not water-soluble.

At the same time, Osborne and Mendel in New Haven were carrying out almost identical experiments to those of Hopkins and of McCollum and Davis. Animals fed synthetic diets in which lard was the only source of fat grew for a while, but then growth stopped, and after a few weeks the animals began to lose weight and die. Adding milk or butter to the synthetic diet always led to recovery. It was the fat component of milk that mattered (9).

Most historians of vitamin research credit McCollum with the discovery of vitamin A. Whereas Hopkins went on to other projects, McCollum persisted in his studies on the trace nutrient in milk, which he initially named "fat-soluble A" (the name was soon changed to "vitamin A"). McCollum and his student Cornelia Kennedy showed that this substance was different from the "water-soluble B" that cured beriberi (thiamin)

---

5   Animals store large quantities of vitamin A in their livers. Rats can last for three months without dietary vitamin A if they are replete at the beginning of that time. Humans can last longer, at least six months, as recent work with vitamin A supplementation has demonstrated.

(10). But it was Hopkins who had made the earlier observation about the growth-sustaining trace nutrient in milk, and it was he who won a share of the Nobel Prize, together with Eijkman, in 1929.[6]

McCollum's name is associated with vitamins for more reasons than just the early work on vitamin A. In 1917 he was hired by Johns Hopkins University and went on to great achievements there. He showed that vitamin D was different from vitamin A, even though both were present in the livers of animals, and helped establish its role as the vitamin that cured rickets. He was instrumental in identifying that there are several water-soluble "B vitamins," and he helped clarify the roles of several minerals in metabolism.

Great scientists — and McCollum was certainly one — often make contributions that depend on new technology; in some cases, the same scientist who comes up with the technology also uses it to make important contributions. That was true for McCollum, who was the first person to establish a colony of inbred rats for nutritional studies in the United States. When he was hired at the University of Wisconsin in 1907, Mc-Collum investigated how best to feed cattle to get them to produce more milk, work that boosted the success of the dairy industry in Wisconsin. But he wanted to work on other problems in nutrition, and he could see that cattle were not ideal for that purpose — too big, too slow growing, too expensive to maintain. He quickly decided that small animals, such as rats, were essential for progress in nutritional science. The following excerpt from his autobiography describes how he came to introduce this important technology to American nutritional research; it also illustrates how homey and simple the conditions for research were early in the 20th century (11):

> A few days later, on Sunday morning when I was at the laboratory, Dr. Babcock [the chair of his department] came in . . . to get his mail. I told him of my idea for a nutrition project using small animals and simplified diets. He was highly enthusiastic. He said

---

6   It isn't clear that Hopkins deserved a share of the Nobel Prize ahead of McCollum. But it would have been impossible to include Hopkins, McCollum, Osborne, and Mendel (in addition to Eijkman) in 1929, since only three individuals can share a given prize in one year. Hopkins made many other contributions to science, but the prize is not meant to be a "lifetime achievement" award.

that the Dean had entered the building a hundred yards in advance of him and was in his office. "Let's go and tell him about it." So we went downstairs, and he led the way into the presence of H. L. Russell. Dr. Babcock told him that I had just outlined an interesting nutrition project which he wanted him to hear about. Then he asked me to tell the Dean of my ideas. I did this in about ten minutes. I explained why only small animals were suitable for the purpose and suggested that I be permitted to develop a rat colony to provide the animals needed.

Dean Russell listened with ill-concealed irritation. When I stopped talking he had the answer on the tip of his tongue. It was "no." We were to experiment with economically valuable animals. The rat was a pest to farmers. If it ever got noised about that we were using federal and state funds to feed rats we should be in disgrace and could never live it down.

Next morning Dr. Babcock came to my laboratory. He sat longer than usual before saying anything. Then he said: "I think the Dean is all wrong in his pronouncement on your new project. I think we should go ahead and do it anyway." I was an instructor in agricultural chemistry drawing a salary of twelve hundred dollars a year. I was not expected to determine policies of the college or experiment station. This I knew very well. But I also knew that everyone about the College and Experiment Station deferred to Dr. Babcock.

. . .

I proceeded at once to make some cages for my rats. I needed some quarter-inch mesh wire screen for this purpose and placed on Hart's desk a requisition for two dollars' worth of this material [Hart was the station chief]. He declined to sign the paper, and so I spent two dollars of my twelve hundred dollar salary to buy the wire screen.

I knew that the old horse barn on the Station farm was infested with rats. On a Saturday afternoon I devoted about two hours to driving the animals out from under the plank floor and into a box-trap. It was similar to the one which my brother and I had made to clear our farmyard of rats when we were little boys. I poured out of the trap into a grain bag seventeen wild gray rats and carried them to the basement of Agricultural Hall and distributed them in my cages.

I soon learned that these rats were too wild, too much alarmed, and too savage to be satisfactory for breeding and experimental work. So I bought for six dollars a dozen young albino rats from a pet-stock dealer in Chicago and paid for them myself. This was the foundation stock of my colony. In January, 1908, I started my first experiment.

In addition to the problems McCollum notes about his ill-fated attempt to use trapped wild rats, it soon became evident that having a more uniform genetic background for animal studies, as provided by inbred albino rats, markedly improved the quality of experimental data because it removed the variability of genetics. The albino rats he was using were among the increasing number of inbred, genetically homogeneous rats and mice being developed at the time by "mouse fanciers" and pet breeders. The descendants of those animals continue to be used for biomedical research today.

McCollum had his faults and made mistakes. His mistakes were significant because he was an important scientist and people paid attention to him. In addition to being widely admired for his research, his influence was enhanced because he had written a seminal textbook, *The Newer Knowledge of Nutrition*. As one example of an important mistake, he declared that scurvy wasn't caused by a nutritional deficit, because rats didn't suffer from it (rats synthesize their own vitamin C, whereas humans can't). He also added his authoritative voice to the notion that pellagra, a vitamin-deficiency disease that became widespread in the United States early in the 20th century, was due to infection (12). That idea was wrong and impeded progress in curing the disease.

McCollum also exhibited some personal flaws — as described by R. D. Semba, "A cloud of accusations of ethical impropriety and professional misconduct accompanied McCollum's departure from Madison [his move from Wisconsin to Johns Hopkins University in 1917] and was aired in print in the journal *Science*" (13). For one thing, station chief E. B. Hart complained that newly appointed Assistant Professor Harry Steenbock was not able to continue an ongoing study because all of the relevant notebooks had disappeared when McCollum left (14); Steenbock was Mc-Collum's graduate student, and his name will come up again in relation to vitamin D. It irritated the Wisconsin scientists that McCollum had not sufficiently noted Steenbock's contributions to work McCollum subsequently published from Johns Hopkins University, much of which had been carried out in Wisconsin, with Steenbock's participation. In addition, Steenbock's contributions to the famous vitamin A paper of McCollum and Davis had not been acknowledged by co-authorship, which his colleagues thought he deserved. McCollum also engaged in a bizarre act of vandalism when he was leaving Madison; after he had taken the rats he wanted to transport to Johns Hopkins with him, he turned the rest loose. It was two months before Steenbock recaptured all of them. McCollum's rationalization was something along the lines that since he had personally provided the rats, they were his to do with as he chose.

There were more Nobel Prizes for vitamin A-related work after 1929. The Swiss chemist Paul Karrer shared the Chemistry Prize in 1937, in part for determining the chemical structure of vitamin A and its precursor, beta-carotene; his determination of the structure of vitamin A in 1931 was the first for any vitamin. And in 1967, three scientists shared the Prize for Physiology or Medicine for describing the mechanisms of vision, including the role of vitamin A. One of those three was George Wald, who had elucidated the role of vitamin A in visual excitation, as we will explore in the next chapter. Vitamin A has more Nobel Prizes associated with its study than any other vitamin. In his Nobel address in 1937, Karrar made another conceptually important point about vitamins (15): "We may perhaps remember that scarcely ten years have elapsed since the time when many research scientists doubted the material specificity of the vitamins, and were of the opinion that a special state of matter, a special colloidal character, was the cause of the peculiar vitamin effects which had been observed." In other words, as late as 1927, many scientists still thought that vitamins weren't specific, defined chemicals, but rather some kind of aggregated (colloidal) state of matter. Karrer's identification of a precise chemical structure for beta-carotene and vitamin A put these ideas to rest.

The term "vitamin" resulted from a faulty assumption by one of Hopkins' friends, the Polish scientist Casimir Funk. Funk was also trying to identify the trace nutrients that he believed were necessary for life. At one point he thought that he had discovered the nature of the anti-beriberi substance (he was mistaken). Funk concluded that just as some of the amino acids found in proteins were essential in the diet because humans can't produce them, there were also other required trace organic compounds. He reasoned that these essential trace nutrients, like the essential amino acids, would be amines, chemicals that are derived from ammonia, so he grouped them under the name "vital amines." He was right about the existence of essential organic micronutrients but wrong about their chemical nature (most are not amines). A certain awkwardness in the naming of the emerging materials — Hopkins' "accessory factors of the diet," Funk's "vital amines," and McCollum's "fat-soluble A" and "water-soluble B" — led to the suggestion that these materials be called "vitamins" (16). At the time, there was vitamin A (fat-soluble), vitamin B (water-soluble), and vitamin C (which prevented scurvy). It would soon become evident that some of these designations comprised several different chemical entities, and the list of vitamin names was about to be lengthened considerably, eventually to the 13 that are today considered essential for human life.

The swirling and sometimes confusing circumstances around the discovery and definition of vitamin A, which continued for years until its chemical structure was determined, were not unusual during the "golden age" of vitamin discovery. Hopkins had unconsciously repeated the earlier (and admittedly somewhat obscured) studies of von Bunge and Pekelharing; McCollum, Osborne, and Mendel had repeated and extended Hopkins' own observations. Others took up the work, and it was soon found that vitamin A is a mixture of closely related, interconvertible compounds. Some are found in plants, some only in animals. But as Hopkins stated in his 1929 Nobel address, we can't attribute the discovery of vitamin A— or, indeed, of most vitamins — to a single person or event.

Vitamin discovery: a many-faceted enterprise

Vitamin A is stored in the livers of animals, together with vitamin D. The latter prevents rickets, a debilitating disease that was described hundreds of years ago as the failure in babies and young children to build strong bones and to thrive. It can lead to lifelong problems of weak bones, malformed ribs, and, in severe cases, death. Because rickets became more prevalent in Europe around the time of the industrial revolution, some thought it was an inevitable condition of modernization, characteristic of industrialized societies in general, one not found in primitive societies "living naturally" (17). The more concrete interpretation, put forward as early as 1822 — that a lack of sunlight was responsible for rickets (18, 19) — was consistent with the effects of the movement of large numbers of rural people into sunless, smoke-beclouded cities during the industrial revolution. But this insight didn't solve the problem, because people had to live in the cities to work. The incidence of rickets increased as industrialization intensified. Between 1901 and 1908, a German physician determined that 90% of children who died before age four in the city of Dresden showed evidence of rickets. Epidemic levels were also seen in parts of the United States during the late 19th and early 20th centuries; estimates of its prevalence in poor inner-city children in America ranged as high as 50% during the first two decades of the 20th century.

Although a lack of sunlight was suspected as a cause of rickets, some physicians' experiences led them to conclude that cod liver oil could prevent it. This was partly based on observations of people living in fishing villages in Scotland, Scandinavia, and the Netherlands, who gave their children cod liver oil, apparently believing that it would prevent rickets. As early as 1824, cod liver oil was prescribed in some places to improve children's health.

A French doctor named Trousseau agreed with this notion and in 1861 also noted that a lack of exposure to the sun predisposed children to develop rickets. He thought that cod liver oil could help prevent rickets, although this insight was weakened by the fact that some batches of cod liver oil didn't work. Trousseau had, in fact, correctly implicated both sunshine and certain oils as important "rickets-preventing" (anti-rachitic) factors. What could these two completely different agents have in common? Or was it just coincidence? The answer to that question, and the identification of the anti-rachitic factor, led to the development of a simple industrial process that overcame vitamin D deficiency and was one of the most profound success stories of the vitamin hunters (19). Like so much of the important work in vitamin discovery, it was a success forged from synergistic work in clinical medicine and laboratory research.

In Austria and Germany, the recurring idea that sunshine could alleviate rickets had led to the practice of placing afflicted infants on balconies in the sun. A physician in Berlin, Kurt Huldschinsky, wondered whether artificial ultraviolet (UV) light might also, like sunlight, combat rickets. He found that it worked and reported this success in 1919. A couple of years later, a British doctor named Harriette Chick obtained essentially the same result, apparently unaware of Huldschinsky's earlier success; she was working in a hospital in Vienna, Austria, and the institution was too poor, after World War I, to subscribe to the journal in which Huldschinsky had described his results (20). Again, as in the work of Hopkins, von Bunge, Eijkman, and Pekelharing, lack of communication meant that important results were confirmed by being discovered more than once.

Chick was a remarkable person (21). After earning a doctorate in bacteriology at University College, in London, she became in 1905 the first woman to get a position at the Lister Institute for medical research.[7] Vienna was particularly hard hit by the aftermaths of World War I, and the British scientists wanted to study diseases related to poor nutrition there. In 1919, Chick travelled to Vienna to help set up studies using cod liver oil and other kinds of fat to treat rachitic children. She had some success, but

---

7   The Lister Institute, which began in 1891, found itself desperately short of funds early in its life and was rescued by a donation from the Guinness family, of beer fame. The association between the brewer and the institute remains to this day.

a confounding factor in interpreting her results was that even the "control group" of children, those not being treated with cod liver oil, seemed to improve during the summer. After further study, she identified sunlight as the factor responsible for their seasonal improvement. The success of two very different treatments for treating rickets — a fat-soluble nutrient and UV light — remained a puzzle, but not for long.

Vitamin D, like vitamin A, is fat-soluble. Both are found in animal livers, which are fat-rich. For a time early in the 20th century, the effects seen with fat-soluble factors were thought to be due to a single agent. It was Hopkins who showed, in 1920, that the "accessory food factor" necessary for rats to thrive, and present in butter (i.e., vitamin A), was destroyed by heating the butter in air. Two years later, McCollum used Hopkins' technique to destroy the growth-sustaining properties of cod liver oil (which are due to vitamin A) and found that this did not interfere with its ability to prevent rickets in rats (22). Vitamin A was not the anti-rachitic factor; another fat-soluble factor was responsible. We know this factor to be vitamin D.

The years 1923–4 were important in the story of vitamin D. Three different research groups found that the effect of UV light on bone development was more subtle and complicated than expected (19). Rats made rachitic by being deprived of fat-soluble micronutrients (i.e., by being starved of vitamin D) were treated with UV light, just as Huldschinsky and Chick had done a few years earlier with children. This was a reversal of the usual flow of discovery, which begins in laboratory animals and is followed by application to humans. The UV treatment of the rachitic rats worked, confirming yet again that when it comes to nutrition, humans and rats often aren't that different. To further analyze this result, the scientists removed one rachitic rat from a cage and then UV-irradiated its partner. They then placed the first rat back into the cage and found, to their surprise, that its rickets was cured, along with that of its irradiated littermate. The next step was to remove *both* rats, irradiate the cage with UV, and then put the rats back in it. Again, the pre-existing rickets went away. This looked like voodoo, but a rational explanation was soon found;

UV irradiation — even in traces of food, or feces in the cage, or the saw-dust on the floor — was enough to prevent or cure rickets (23).

Harry Steenbock may have been short-changed for his contributions to McCollum's work, but now he and his colleagues came to prominence following their own observations on the ability of UV irradiation to cure rickets in rats (24). The Wisconsin group made the practical discovery that irradiation of many foods containing fats also prevented rickets. They filed a patent for producing vitamin D in milk by irradiating it with UV light, and this technology more or less brought rickets to an end in the modern world.

The irradiation process discovered in Steenbock's laboratory led to the creation of the Wisconsin Alumni Research Foundation (WARF), designed to look after the intellectual property generated by its faculty. At the time, the usual procedure for university research with practical poten-tial was to sell it to an interested commercial entity. There were certainly companies willing to pay a lot of money for the rights to Steenbock's vitamin D enrichment discovery, including Quaker Oats, who offered a million dollars (equivalent to about $14 million today). But a group of nine Wisconsin alumni wanted to do something more imaginative and profitable. Using their own money, they set up WARF as an agency whol-ly owned by the university, to maintain control of the irradiation patent, which would be licensed to commercial interests. That was prescient as well as very unusual at the time. Their vision was that future inventions would also be taken up by WARF and managed by the university for prof-it, and this is what happened. (One of its greatest successes was the dis-covery of an anti-clotting drug that they called "Warfarin." It remains the most commonly used drug to prevent blood clotting.) Under the terms of each arrangement, the inventor would get 20% of the gross royalty reve-nue and WARF would keep the rest, from which it would pay the filing costs for patent applications and the legal costs for protecting the intellec-tual property. Any additional earnings would go to benefit research on the campus. So, WARF paid for and maintained the patent on the vitamin D process and licensed it to Quaker Oats and other companies. By the time that this patent expired, WARF had earned eight million dollars from it, equivalent to around $100 million today.[8]

It took further years of work to understand the relationship between UV irradiation, cod liver oil, and vitamin D. UV light causes a chemical reaction in skin or food that converts a steroid precursor to vitamin D.[9] Codfish accumulate the vitamin in their livers, accounting for the anti-rachitic properties of cod liver oil. A remarkable thing about vitamin D is that its production from a steroid precursor is a chemical reaction directly induced by UV light from sunlight or a lamp. This reaction produced vitamin D in the residual materials in the cages of the rachitic rats, and it produces the vitamin D in our skin during exposure to a source of UV light.

The role of human disease in vitamin discovery continued in the early years of the 20th century, when a mysterious epidemic arose in the United States, centred in the southern states (25). The symptoms were soon identified as being due to pellagra, a disease that was familiar in Spain and northern Italy but little understood. It was usually associated with poverty. Beginning with a few isolated cases at the turn of the century, there were ever more cases and deaths in America, and by the time the epidemic ended, around 1935, there had been an estimated three million cases and 100,000 deaths. (These numbers were undoubtedly underestimates; authorities were reluctant to report the actual embarrassing numbers of cases in their jurisdictions.) Notably, the disease was most often observed in "confined" populations, reminiscent of the beriberi experience: orphanages, prisons, and — particularly — insane asylums. The symptoms of pellagra could be summarized by four "Ds": dermatitis, diarrhoea, dementia, and death.

The occurrence of pellagra induced the kind of fear and irrationality that in later years accompanied the AIDS epidemic. The most damaging conclusion about its cause was that pellagra was infectious, an opinion also held by the great vitamin hunter E. V. McCollum. A commission

---

8   The success of WARF continues. In the Fall of 2015, a Wisconsin jury ordered Apple Inc. to pay WARF $234 million for patent infringement related to technology used in its iPhone and iPad chips. Based on its success over the decades, WARF continues to pour millions of dollars into research at the university.

9   Vitamin D from the diet or induced by UV light requires activation in the liver before it can work.

appointed to study the disease concluded, on the basis of house-to-house surveys in afflicted cotton mill districts of the southern United States, that there was no connection between pellagra and diet, and that it occurred almost exclusively in people who lived next door to another person with pellagra. The first conclusion was simply wrong, the second obvious and uninformative: poor people live together in areas called slums. At the time, the paradigm that epidemic diseases always had microbial causes still held sway. Whenever diet was brought up as a possible cause of pellagra, it was angrily dismissed; in the South, the embarrassing idea that poverty was causing the epidemic was too much to bear for a damaged society still sensitive from the affront of the Civil War. Anyone trying to find a solution other than infection was given short shrift.

Then, in 1914, Dr. Joseph Goldberger appeared on the scene. Goldberger was an officer of the US Public Health Service, a Jewish New Yorker from the Lower East Side, and before that an immigrant from Hungary. His parents had managed to put him through medical school, from which he graduated at 21. But he was unsuccessful in obtaining a position as a private physician. After several other attempts at finding a job, he wrote a competitive examination for the Public Health Service, got the highest score in the country, and subsequently spent his career with that organization. Goldberger quickly arrived at the opinion that pellagra was not in any way infectious. Health care professionals who treated victims never got sick, nor did the staff at institutions whose inmates were at high risk. Another clue came from orphanages: children below the age of six or over 16 seldom got pellagra. Those under six were being given milk in their diets, and those over 16 were required to work, so they were fed diets enriched in other ways (such as with more meat). Goldberger concluded that a dietary deficit was probably responsible for pellagra and soon was able to set up studies that showed this was the case. He solicited federal funds to improve the diet in one asylum, and no new cases arose; when the funds ran out, the old diet was resumed, and pellagra came back. He then approached the governor of Mississippi to ask to have a group of prisoners on one of the state's prison farms take part in a further test of his ideas about pellagra. The 12 men were promised that their sentences would be shortened if they participated (and survived). Six of the men were fed a diet similar to that of poor people in the state, and the others were given in addition collard greens and cabbage. The study had to be terminated when the first group came down with pellagra and begged to be taken out of it. As a final test of the infectious disease hypothesis, Goldberger exposed himself and his fellow scientists to bodily substances from pellagra victims, without ill effect other than some cases of nausea and diarrhoea.

The cause of pellagra was an absence of the vitamin called nicotinic acid, now known by the less tobacco-redolent name of niacin. In almost every case, the victims were poor people on diets in which most of their calories came from corn. Corn itself wasn't the problem: Amerindians living in the South and in central America had depended heavily on corn but didn't seem to have suffered much, if at all, from pellagra. There appeared to be two reasons for this difference. First, Indian culture called for the treatment of corn with lime water, which is alkaline and increases the availability of the niacin present in corn. Secondly, in 1900, just before the pellagra epidemic started, the Beall Company, of Decatur, Illinois, proudly announced the invention of the "Beall Degerminator," which efficiently removed the bran components of corn during grinding to corn meal. This gave the corn better storage properties, since the fat was removed. Unfortunately, so was niacin. The cornmeal kept better on the shelf but was a poor source of nutrition. A further clue was that people working in factories, who bought commercial, degerminated cornmeal, were at high risk for pellagra, while those who were agrarian, grew their own corn, and used it un-degerminated were generally not. The situation has clear parallels with the beriberi saga in Indonesia.[10]

The solution to pellagra was simple: niacin quickly corrected the deficiency. Yeast was a good and inexpensive source of niacin, as well as other vitamins of the B group, such as thiamin and riboflavin. Pellagra was eliminated in the United States by the 1940s. Like the effect of rice polishing in the Dutch East Indies, which removed the bran and thereby thiamin, the modern "improvement" of corn milling led to a serious health problem. Eijkman would probably have nodded in sympathy.

---

10 In its current ads, Beall still refers to the Degerminator as "an outstanding discovery."

Although a clear grasp of the existence, nature, and significance of vitamins only began about a hundred years ago, there were clues earlier, sometimes much earlier. An iconic story concerning the early history of vitamins is that of British sailors who suffered from scurvy. After a few months at sea, scurvy could bring a healthy man down with ulcerated gums, teeth that fell out, anemia, and sudden death due to rupture of a major blood vessel. The problem of long sea voyages was brought to particular prominence by the death rate on a circumnavigation of the world that ended in 1740: of the 1,900 men who had started on the voyage, 1,400 apparently died of scurvy. The Scottish physician and ship's doctor James Lind decided to study this condition on voyages of his own naval vessel, and in 1747 he began what was probably the world's first clinical trial. His hypothesis was that scurvy was caused by decay in the body, which could be stopped by acid. He divided 12 sailors suffering from scurvy into six groups, each of which was given the same diet, with supplementation as follows: each day, the first group received a quart of cider, the second, 25 drops of vitriol (sulphuric acid), the third, vinegar, the fourth half a pint of seawater, the fifth, two oranges and one lemon, and the last a spicy paste plus barley water. Group five, the fortunate ones receiving the citrus fruits, had almost recovered from their scurvy after five days, when the citrus fruit ran out; then they began to go downhill again. Group one showed slight improvement, while all the rest were as sick as ever. A few years later Lind published a description of this experiment, but it was almost completely ignored. Lind's notion was that scurvy was caused by poorly digested and putrefying food in the body, a process stopped by something in citrus fruit. He never provided a clear statement of the benefit of citrus fruit, and it took until almost the end of the 18th century before citrus fruits (lemons and limes) were incorporated into the diets of sailors, bringing scurvy under control.

Although citrus fruits were known to contain vitamin C, which prevented scurvy, the chemical nature of vitamin C was not determined until 1931. A number of laboratories were working to isolate vitamin C from lemon juice, beginning in the early 1920s. The work was painstaking: biochemical techniques were still primitive, and measuring the biological activity of vitamin C was a long and tedious process. The only known biological activity was its ability to prevent scurvy. By that time, the nutrition of rats was considered quite a good model for human nutrition in many ways, but a need for vitamin C was not one of them, because rats, unlike humans, can synthesize their own vitamin C (this led McCollum to his mistaken notion that vitamin C wasn't really a vitamin). But guinea pigs, which are larger, more costly, and generally less convenient to work with than rats, do share with humans a need for vitamin C in their diet, so researchers attempting to isolate vitamin C in the laboratory used guinea pigs. The detection of vitamin C was a cumbersome process. Animals fed a diet devoid of vitamin C (somewhat along the lines of Hopkins' early work using vitamin A-deficient diets with rats) would die after about three weeks. Giving them vitamin C in the form of lemon extracts would save them. But the guinea pigs had to be observed for another four weeks or so, to ensure they were really alright. So each experiment with vitamin C in an extract or a semi-purified preparation would take up to 60 days and involve a dozen or more guinea pigs. Not surprisingly, progress in purifying vitamin C was glacially slow. A number of groups pursued this avenue of work and by 1931 had achieved some hard-won success.

Purification of vitamin C from a natural product (lemons) didn't provide much information about its chemical nature.[11] The scientists knew that vitamin C was acidic, that it did not contain any nitrogen, and that it was very potent — milligram quantities could save a guinea pig from death by scurvy. Determination of its chemical structure, though, came from work that the "purifiers" never discussed in their publications, which was not surprising, since it bore no apparent connection to vitamin C. That line of work was being pursued by a Hungarian scientist named Albert Szent-Györgyi. Born in 1893, Szent-Györgyi entered medical school in 1911 but had his studies interrupted in 1914 by World War I. He served as an army medic on the Italian and Russian fronts (Hungary was allied with Germany) and was rewarded for his valorous service with

---

11 Determining the chemical nature of a natural product such as vitamin C, in addition to being important information in itself, is essential for it to be produced synthetically, which in the case of vitamin C has yielded a cheap, essentially unlimited supply.

a Silver Medal. However, he was fed up with war, and to end his service, he carefully shot himself in the arm, claimed the wound was received in battle, and was sent home to finish medical school. He then began a long series of training and research experiences in various places: Berlin, Hamburg, Leiden, and Groningen, these last two being in the Netherlands.

During Szent-Györgyi's early research career, it was already clear that living organisms generate the energy they need by oxidation — foodstuffs such as carbohydrate or fat are combusted ("burned") in the presence of oxygen, producing heat and energy. This is why our "human engine" needs a certain number of calories of food each day. That food can be burned in the flame of a candle in an uncontrolled way, or it can be oxidized in the body under tightly controlled conditions of energy metabolism to generate the same energy. Oxidation was also behind other biological processes, and Szent-Györgyi recognized that the study of biological oxidation was an exciting research area.

In the early 1920s, while still on his peripatetic adventure in research, Szent-Györgyi became interested in the oxidation–reduction properties of the adrenal gland. He knew that people whose adrenal gland secreted too little of one of its hormones had a condition called "Addison's disease," with one of its effects being a brown colouration of the skin.[12] He wondered whether that skin condition might be related to the browning that occurs when some fruits are cut and left out in the air, which is due to oxidation. In other words, perhaps by studying the browning of cut fruit he could find out something useful about Addison's disease. This was a red herring and led to no useful information about the adrenal gland. But he did find that the adrenal gland contained a reducing substance, an antioxidant, and decided to study it.

Although his early research provided some interesting observations, by 1926 Szent-Györgyi was in despair. He couldn't find support for his work, job prospects were bleak, and he couldn't see any way forward. But in Stockholm, at what he thought would be his last scientific meeting, he was astonished to hear his work on the adrenal gland praised by none other than Sir Frederick Gowland Hopkins, a god of the research world.

---

12   President John F. Kennedy had Addison's disease.

He introduced himself to Hopkins, and in 1927, at Hopkins' invitation, he arrived in Cambridge on a well-supported research fellowship.

There, he continued his interest in the reducing (anti-oxidizing) factor from the adrenal gland. It was difficult to isolate, given the primitive state of biochemical purification technology at that time. He had to carry out a series of precipitations of the antioxidant using various organic solvents and then finally crystallize it. But the biggest problem was supply: the starting material, bovine adrenal glands, was scarce. The Mayo Foundation came to his rescue by offering to bring him to the United States to work with slaughterhouse material, an abundant source of adrenal glands. After a year in America, he returned to Cambridge with 50 grams of his reducing compound. He applied various chemical tests and determined that he was dealing with a "hexuronic acid" — that is, a weak organic acid with six carbon atoms in its chemical structure, somewhat similar to glucose (26).

In 1928 Szent-Györgyi was invited to return to Hungary, to the University of Szeged, to head up biomedical research there. He did so in January 1931, with his small, precious supply of hexuronic acid in his suitcase. Although it didn't help explain much about the adrenal gland's function, the new compound looked interesting from a chemical point of view, and Szent-Györgyi sought a more copious supply of it in the plant world. It was present in, among other places, oranges and cabbage. But the mother lode turned out to be a fruit that was peculiarly apt to his Hungarian location: paprika peppers. From these he was quickly able to isolate pounds of his hexuronic acid, and he just as quickly distributed it to various research centres around the world to see what anyone could make of it. He sent one sample to chemistry professor Norman Howarth at Birmingham University in England to study its structure. Haworth, who was widely acknowledged to be the world's most outstanding carbohydrate chemist, determined its structure in 1933 and a year later reported its synthesis in the laboratory.

But even before Szent-Györgyi discovered that paprika peppers were a great source of his hexuronic acid, when he still had only milligram quantities of it, something quite astonishing happened. One of the groups of scientists patiently purifying vitamin C was at the University of Pittsburgh, in the United States, led by a man named Charles Glen King. In 1931, his group had finally isolated and crystallized vitamin C, the anti-scurvy agent, from lemon juice (27). One of the students working in King's laboratory was a Hungarian, Joseph Svirbely. Svirbely was directly involved in measuring vitamin C levels using guinea pigs, so he was intimately familiar with this technology. He had contributed to published work on the purification of vitamin C in King's laboratory. In the autumn of 1931, Svirbely received an invitation from Szent-Györgyi to join him in Szeged, which he did. Until then, Szent-Györgyi had been reluctant to engage in animal experiments with his hexuronic acid, as he still had only milligram quantities of it (the discovery about paprika was still two years in the future). But Svirbely was expert at using guinea pigs, and Szent-Györgyi had a hunch that his hexuronic acid, which had reducing properties, might be related to vitamin C, the antioxidant that had been purified in King's laboratory. Even if the two were not identical, hexuronic acid might have an effect on vitamin C-deprived animals. So he handed Svirbely his precious supply of hexuronic acid, and the result was of historic importance: hexuronic acid cured scurvy in guinea pigs.

Svirbely informally communicated this remarkable result to his old research supervisor, King, who was shocked, to say the least. He immediately sent a communication to the prestigious American journal *Science*, claiming that he knew his vitamin C was Szent-Györgyi's hexuronic acid (28). That paper contained no proof of this assertion — in fact, no data at all; his claim was based on his knowledge of Svirbely's results through personal communication. When he heard that King was publishing this, Szent-Györgyi immediately fired off a publication of his own to the equally prestigious British journal *Nature* (29). This paper contained the data showing that hexuronic acid cured scurvy in guinea pigs. Szent-Györgyi asserted that the striking similarity between vitamin C and hexuronic acid had long been evident to him, although he did not indicate where he had previously expressed this idea. He repeated that assertion when he won the Nobel Prize for Physiology or Medicine in 1937. King was not included in that honour, much to his chagrin, but in favour of Szent-Györgyi's claim to primacy was that he knew the chemical composition, and that by 1937 the structure of his hexuronic acid and its anti-scurvy activity had been demonstrated in his laboratory. On the other hand, King had been working on vitamin C the whole time and had isolated it in near-pure form.

As more copious quantities of hexuronic acid became available, its biological activities were tested thoroughly and found to mimic all of the effects of vitamin C in curing scurvy. In addition, Howarth in Birmingham determined its chemical structure and in 1934 its chemical synthesis. Scientists studying natural products consider the proof of the nature of such materials to involve two distinct steps: analysis and synthesis. Analysis of purified material provides the scientist with information about its structure, but there is a potential hitch. Until the material can be synthesized from simple starting materials in the laboratory, it is possible that the material being analyzed is not responsible for the biological activity observed — a highly potent contaminant, present in trace amounts, could be the active component. But synthesis settles the argument, and Howarth had done both analysis and synthesis. In 1937, Szent-Györgyi won a Nobel Prize for discovering vitamin C, and Howarth shared a Prize (in Chemistry) for his contributions to carbohydrate chemistry, including the work on vitamin C. Charles Glen King never won a Nobel Prize, but he made many contributions to nutritional science throughout the rest of his career (both King and Szent-Györgyi were not yet 40 when vitamin C was solved). For his part, Szent-Györgyi became an extraordinarily creative investigator of biological oxidation and related metabolic activities.

The discovery of vitamins continued into the mid-20th century, and 13 have been identified that are essential for human life. Since the mid-1930s, purification methods have become much more powerful, and the identification of the vitamins discovered since then has proceeded more rapidly than during the "golden age" of vitamin discovery. The names of most of them are recognizable from articles about nutrition in the popular press or from the labels on packaged food. Other animal species can have other needs, or may not need all of the human-required vitamins; for example, rats and many other animal species don't need vitamin C in their diet. But there are enough overlaps that animals can serve as surrogates for studying vitamins essential to human life. The other approach to vitamin discovery was clinical observation and intervention, of which Eijkman's work in Java is an early example — the observation that first chickens and then humans whose diets consisted almost entirely of polished rice suffered from beriberi was the starting point for the discovery of the B vitamins. A later example of clinical observation leading to vitamin discovery is related to folic acid.

In terms of its chemical structure, folic acid is one of the more complex vitamins. Its discovery began in India (30). An English doctor in the 1920s and 1930s was studying a form of anemia that poor Indian women were experiencing during pregnancy. This study was unusual for at least two reasons — that such work was being done in India at all, and that the doctor doing them was a woman, Lucy Wills. Wills was a beneficiary of late Victorian reformers who had campaigned for the right of women to be educated in the professions. She came from the upper middle class and was of the generation and class of women in Britain who sought to achieve at the highest levels. (Harriette Chick, who helped discover vitamin D with her studies in post-war Vienna, was another.) Wills received what was, at the time, a progressive and radical education for a woman. She obtained a double first-class honours in Botany and Geology at Cambridge, a remarkable achievement for anyone. After a year in South Africa, she entered the London School of Medicine for Women, part of the University of London, which was the first medical school in Britain to train women physicians. Wills opted for medical research and began to learn about the metabolic problems of pregnancy. She became a pathologist at the same teaching hospital where she trained.

In 1928, at age 40 and in response to a request by a senior colleague, Wills began her most important work, the study of anemia in pregnancy in India, which she pursued for five years. She found that it was particularly prevalent in poor women in Bombay, especially Muslims, who ate almost no fruits or vegetables and often died during pregnancy. Her approach included subjecting laboratory rats to the same diets, and these also died during pregnancy. Consumption of yeast prevented the condition in the rats and was soon saving the lives of patients. The nutrient missing in their diets was named the "Wills Factor." It was isolated in 1941 and determined to be folic acid, vitamin B9, a water-soluble micronutrient that humans (and rats) cannot produce (Wills was not involved in this later work). Since 1998, Canada and the USA have required that enriched breads and other grain products contain supplemental folic acid, which has reduced the incidence of birth defects such as spina bifida.[13]

There was a dearth of young men in England after the end of World War I — too many had been slaughtered — and perhaps because of this, Wills never married. Or perhaps she enjoyed her life in medicine too much to risk losing it by the wrong kind of marriage. She obviously had an independent way about her, and she was viewed by contemporaries as having no patience for laziness and foolishness. A former student referred to her as "naturally aristocratic but anti-establishment" (31). In retirement, she returned to her student interest in botany and created a botanical garden.

Another vitamin important for the prevention of anemia, in addition to folic acid (vitamin B9), is cyanocobalamine (vitamin B12). A deficiency of this vitamin, which has several chemical forms, can lead to pernicious anemia. It has the most complex chemical structure of any of the vitamins. This structure was determined in the 1950s using a new and powerful physical-chemical methodology called X-ray crystallography. In this technique, the molecule of interest is crystallized in a regular crystal form, through which parallel beams of X-rays are directed. Deflection of the beam by the atoms of the crystallized molecule is measured on photographic film, and that information can be used to determine its three-dimensional structure. Because X-rays have very short wavelengths, they can "see" the atoms in a molecule, something that longer wavelength radiation, such as visible light, cannot do. A feature that made vitamin B12 amenable to structural determination is that it contains an atom of cobalt. Determining a complex structure like that of vitamin B12 using X-ray crystallography requires a sort of molecular reference point, generally an unusually dense atom of a metal, located at a precise point in

---

13 Spina bifida is one example of birth defects due to improper development of the spinal column and brain during pregnancy. Other effects of folic acid deficiency include anemia.

the structure. The heavy metal deflects the incoming X-rays much more strongly than the carbon, hydrogen, and oxygen atoms that make up the rest of the molecule, and that perturbation helps the crystallographer interpret the data to determine the chemical structure. The cobalt atom in vitamin B12 is just such a reference point. When its three-dimensional structure was determined in 1956, by Professor Dorothy Crowfoot Hodgkin at Oxford University, it was the most complicated structure solved to that time (Crowfoot Hodgkin won a Nobel Prize in 1964 for solving the structures of a number of natural products, including vitamin B12).

Humans need 13 vitamins, which they mostly obtain from their diets or, in the case of vitamin D, from ambient ultraviolet light. Each has its own story of discovery. A number of them are grouped together as B vitamins, which are generally water-soluble. (One of the B vitamins, riboflavin, is actually poorly soluble in water.) The B vitamin biotin is only a borderline dietary requirement for humans — deficiency due to poor diet is practically unheard of, because intestinal bacteria produce it. Pantothenic acid (vitamin B5) and pyridoxine (B6), as well as a few others, are also rarely deficient in humans. But even if deficiency is rare, all of the vitamins are essential to life. For example, each of the B vitamins plays an essential role in metabolism, where they are co-factors for the enzymes that carry out the chemical reactions of living cells. Cells cannot function without them. But because they are present in many foods, deficiencies of some vitamins are rare.

The importance of vitamin discovery is underscored by the number of Nobel Prizes associated with it. Beginning with Eijkman and Hopkins, 16 prizes were awarded for the discovery or study of vitamins between 1929 and 1964. Some of those awards were for Chemistry, some were for Physiology or Medicine. Unfortunately, some major contributions were never rewarded with a Nobel Prize, although they were just as meritorious. Osborne, Mendel, and McCollum (for their work on vitamin A), among others, probably belong in this group.

The discovery of vitamins was a complicated and sometimes messy endeavour, but it was completed by 1950. Each of the 13 vitamins needed by humans was chemically identified and one or more functions determined.

But as work on vitamins continued, it became clear that the first function identified for a particular vitamin often isn't the only one that matters. This was particularly true for vitamin A, which had become known as the "vision vitamin." Vitamin A is indeed essential for vision, but that is only part of the story, and in terms of human health, not the most important part. The vitamin's importance in maintaining the immune system and regulating the growth and development of the body have emerged as its most important roles in human health. Without vitamin A, life itself is under threat, as Alfred Sommer discovered in Indonesia. Blindness is not a direct threat to life, but a crippled immune system can be. The reasons vitamin A is so important to human health are a direct result of its complicated biological functions, as we will explore in the next chapter. Vitamin A is the most complex of the vitamins, something not realized until long after it had been identified. The study of these complexities continues to provide, and solve, mysteries in biomedical science and helps explain its effects on human biology.

CHAPTER 3

The Science of Vitamin A

Vitamin A has several chemical and physical forms

Our understanding of the activities of vitamin A has changed profoundly over the past 50 years. Its role in vision was well understood before, but we now realize that it plays a critical role in a long list of functions essential for life, including growth and development, resistance to disease, and normal tissue health. These non-vision functions derive from its role as a regulator of gene expression. In fact, the roles of vitamin A in gene regulation and vision have nothing directly to do with each other. This is also true for vitamin D, which is essential for bone health and also affects the expression of several genes, by a mechanism that is unrelated to its direct effects on bone development. The role of vitamin A (and vitamin D) in gene regulation exists only in eukaryotic cells, cells that have a nucleus. The roles of vitamin A in visual function and gene regulation are played by different but closely related chemical forms.

The most abundant form of vitamin A in animals is retinol, and only animal sources of food contain it. This is the form in which vitamin A is stored in the human liver (Figure 1).

Retinol is one form of "preformed vitamin A." To simplify the description of the various forms of vitamin A in the following figures, the core structure identified in Figure 1 appears as "R." Retinol (which we will call R-CH$_2$OH) has an alcohol group at the right-hand end of the carbon chain There are five carbon–carbon double bonds in retinol, arranged as double bonds alternating with single bonds. This is called a "conjugated"

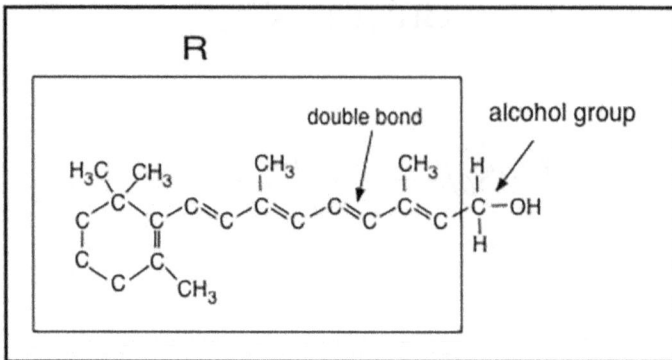

Figure 1. *Retinol. For simplicity, most hydrogen atoms are not shown. One of the five double bonds is identified. The core structure of all forms of vitamin A is the inner boxed section, labeled "R."*

system; this information will become relevant when we discuss some of the activities of vitamin A. The double bond identified in Figure 1 is important for the function of vitamin A during the visual cycle (as will be described a bit later, in Figure 5).

Retinol contains 20 carbon atoms, which is a direct result of how it is synthesized. In natural systems, many complex chemicals, including vitamin A and steroids such as cholesterol, are built from five-carbon units joined together like so many Lego blocks. The five-carbon building blocks, in turn, are created by cellular enzymes from two-carbon units that result from the breakdown (oxidation) of fats. Three of these two-carbon units are stitched together, during which one carbon is lost, forming the five-carbon blocks. These are then used to build complex structures, some of which, like cholesterol and vitamin A, even contain rings. Vitamin A is the result of a synthetic scheme involving four such five-carbon blocks, which yields a structure containing 20 carbon atoms. This kind of synthetic scheme is present in all life forms, including plants and bacteria, although its details vary between organisms.

During digestion, retinol is converted to retinyl esters, which are complexes of retinol and some of the common fatty acids. These are chemically linked to the alcohol group of retinol. Because they are very soluble in fat and insoluble in water, retinyl esters circulate in the blood associated with chylomicron particles. Chylomicrons, one of the blood lipids measured during clinical blood work, transport digested fats. In addition to retinyl esters, they contain "bad" cholesterol, as well as fats, certain proteins, and other fat-soluble materials. Retinyl esters are also the form in which vitamin A is stored in the human body, primarily in the liver. Retinol is released from or stored in the liver to maintain the correct level of vitamin A in the blood. The liver can store a large quantity of vitamin A,[14] meaning that if vitamin A levels are severely depleted, which is periodically the case for millions of children in the developing world, an individual can safely be given a large dose of retinol in a capsule to rebuild the liver's supply of retinyl esters. This is the most common way of providing vitamin A to deficient children.

Plants do not contain retinol or retinyl esters. Those that contain vitamin A, such as orange sweet potatoes, carrots, and spinach, have a different form, called beta-carotene. Beta-carotene is referred to as "provitamin A" and needs to be cleaved into "preformed vitamin A" to be useful to the animal body. It consists essentially of two molecules of preformed vitamin A, joined head-to-head by a double bond (Figure 2).

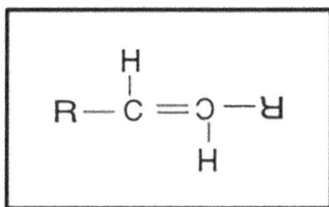

Figure 2. *Beta-carotene. The molecule consists of two of the "R" groups identified in Figure 1, joined by a double bond. In this figure, the two halves of the molecule are upside down with respect to each other to reflect the fact that the molecule is symmetrical (it can be rotated around an axis perpendicular to the page, running through the double bond).*

There is a profound advantage to getting vitamin A from plants in the form of beta-carotene rather than by consuming retinol: while excess retinol can be acutely toxic, it is almost impossible to get an overdose of

---

14 Certain foods — for example, the livers of some animals — contain so much vitamin A that they are toxic for humans; the next chapter describes an example.

beta-carotene. This is because the enzyme that cleaves beta-carotene into retinal in the gut is inhibited by high circulating levels of vitamin A, which automatically slow down the process, preventing an overdose (32, 33).

Beta-carotene as such has no activities in the animal body, aside from being converted to preformed vitamin A. In plants, it has several roles, including increasing the efficiency of photosynthesis and acting as an antioxidant (34). The roles of vitamin A in plants and animals have nothing to do with each other. Plants use beta-carotene for one set of purposes; animals have evolved to use it for others. Although chlorophyll is the most important molecule for absorbing light during photosynthesis, other coloured molecules, or chromophores, increase its efficiency because they absorb different wavelengths than chlorophyll and transfer the energy they absorb to the photosynthetic structures. Beta-carotene is one of these. In addition to being an "antenna" for certain wavelengths of light, it also increases the efficiency of photosynthesis in other, more subtle ways (35). Sunlight can damage molecules in cells; by absorbing some of the sun's energy, beta-carotene acts as a "sunblock." In Fall, when chlorophyll, with its intense green masking colour, disappears, the leaves of some trees reflect the presence of the yellow-orange carotenoids, including beta-carotene. (Some Fall colours are due to other chromophores.) The role of beta-carotene in protecting plant cells against oxidative damage will be described later.

During digestion, beta-carotene is broken down to a form of vitamin A called retinal, which is slightly different from retinol (Figure 3). Retinal and retinol have the same core structure ("R" in Figure 1) and are easily interconverted. The role of vitamin A in vision involves retinal, which is the vitamin's aldehyde form; a little later in this chapter, we will examine a remarkable property of retinal required for vision. The retinal produced during digestion is readily converted to retinol in the gut, and retinol is converted into retinal in the eye's cells responsible for vision.

There is another form of vitamin A, and it's the most important of all in terms of its effects on animal life. This is retinoic acid, also depicted in Figure 3. The series retinol–retinal–retinoic acid represents progressively more oxidized forms of vitamin A. Retinol, an alcohol, is oxidized by cellular enzymes to retinal, an aldehyde, and retinal in turn is converted by oxidation to retinoic acid (Figure 4). The interconversion of retinol and retinal goes in either direction. But the step from retinal to retinoic acid is one-directional; cells have no pathway for the reduction of retinoic acid to retinal.

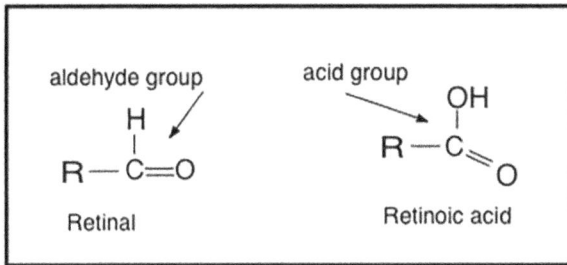

Figure 3. *Retinal and retinoic acid. Retinal is the aldehyde form of vitamin A (indicated by the -al ending). It is produced from beta-carotene during digestion and from retinol in the cells of the eye. Retinoic acid is the form of vitamin A involved in a wide variety of gene regulatory functions.*

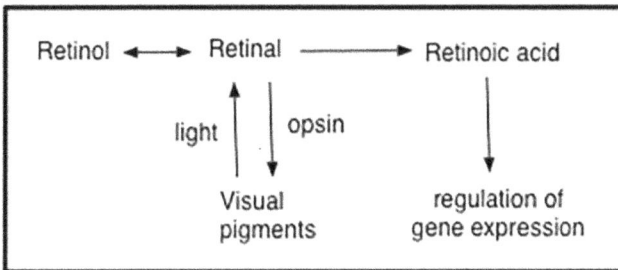

Figure 4. *The interconversion of various forms of vitamin A. The alcohol form (retinol) is interconvertible with the aldehyde form (retinal), but the conversion of retinal to retinoic acid goes in only one direction. The interaction of retinal with opsin in the eye is described in Figure 5.*

A description of the role of vitamin A in the visual cycle in rod cells is shown in Figure 5. It involves both retinol and retinal. A critical feature is that the retinol and retinal molecules undergo a shape change, called isomerization, during the cycle. "All-trans retinol" is depicted in Figure 1 (page 52). The term all-trans refers to the configuration about the double bonds in the molecule; they are all in a "trans" state, and the long tail of the molecule runs in a smooth, slightly curved line. This form of retinol is isomerized to "11-cis retinol" during the visual cycle, as shown in Figure 5. The number "11" refers to the position of the double bond that undergoes isomerization. The 11-cis retinol is oxidized to 11-cis retinal, which forms a linkage with the protein opsin to form rhodopsin, the visual pigment. When the rhodopsin molecule captures a photon of light, the retinal isomerizes to its all-trans form and is released. The opsin protein undergoes a shape change during this event, which initiates a series of biochemical and electrical perturbations in the membrane around it. This activates the photoreceptor cell — the first step in seeing.

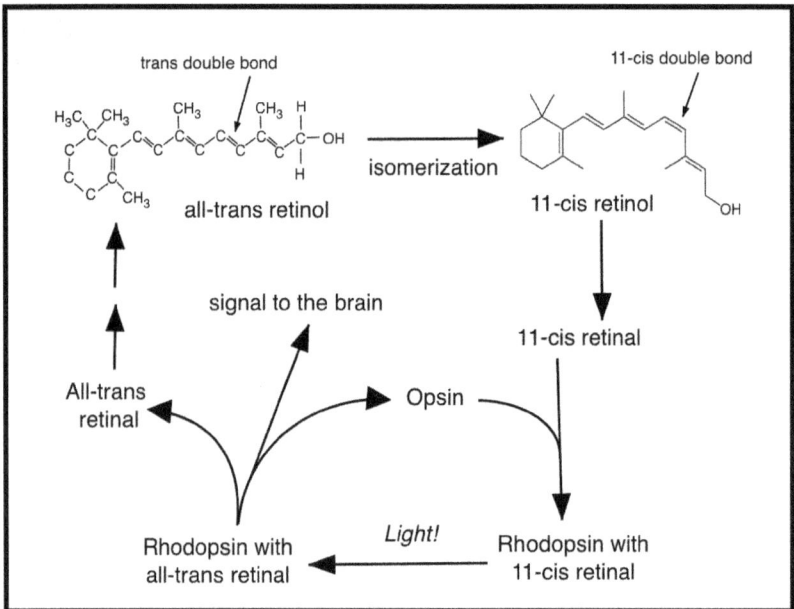

Figure 5. *Vitamin A in the visual cycle. All-trans retinol is the structure shown in Figure 1. It undergoes enzyme-catalyzed isomerization to 11-cis retinol, followed by enzymatic oxidation to 11-cis retinal. (The —CH3 groups in 11-cis retinol are represented by lines.) 11-cis retinal spontaneously associates with the opsin protein to form rhodopsin. Visible light causes the retinal to flip to the all-trans form, which is then released from opsin. Opsin activated by this event alters its shape, leading to visual excitation.*

Rhodopsin, located in the rod cells of the eye, is the visual pigment that responds to low light. A deficit in rhodopsin causes nightblindness during vitamin A deficiency, as we will examine in detail a bit later. In addition to opsin, three other visual proteins bind retinal in the human eye. These are located in different photoreceptors, in the cone cells. The opsins of the cone cells are responsible for colour vision. Combined with retinal, they fire in response to either red, green, or blue light, respectively. Each of these opsins of the cone cells binds the same retinal molecule, more or less as rhodopsin does, but each has its own protein component, and this makes the three visual pigments sensitive to one of the three colours. Working together, the cone opsins reconstitute a colour image in the brain, somewhat as a colour television does with its RGB inputs.

The roles of the different forms of vitamin A in animals can be summarized as follows. Retinol, or "preformed vitamin A," is a storage and distribution form of the vitamin, without any direct effects of its own. It is converted to retinal, the aldehyde form, in cells of the eye, where it combines with visual proteins (opsin for low-light vision, one of the cone cell proteins for colour vision) to form the visual pigments, sensitive to light, that initiate visual events. Retinoic acid is formed from retinal in many types of cells, and its functions are the most complex of any of the forms of vitamin A. These functions, essential to life, will be described in some detail after we delve further into vitamin A's role in vision.

Vitamin A is essential for vision

Most people are aware that vitamin A is important for vision and that a deficiency can lead to "nightblindness" (poor vision at night) or worse. What we know about the activity of retinal in the retina of the eye is consistent with this. A deficiency of retinal causes a loss of rhodopsin in the eye, and night vision suffers. But why isn't daytime, colour vision affected just as much? The answer is that the three retinal-protein complexes responsible for colour vision bind retinal more tightly than opsin does, and generally operate in brighter light. As a result, they are less sensitive to low levels of vitamin A than rhodopsin, which is the first of the visual pigments to be affected by a decline in retinal. Nightblindness is the initial effect of vitamin A deficiency on vision, and it is reversible. But a chronic deficit in vitamin A does eventually affect colour vision too, and the end result of severe vitamin A deficiency is total, irreversible blindness, for reasons that we will examine a bit later.

An elegant description of the results of vitamin A deficiency was provided by the American biologist George Wald in a seminal paper in 1958. Wald was one of the remarkably large number of American scientists who began their lives in New York City as children of poor immigrants or refugees from Europe around the beginning of the 20th century. Wald's mother and father, from Germany and Poland, respectively, lived in Brooklyn in 1906, the year George was born. George was a brilliant young man who altered, or at least augmented, his range of interests frequently throughout an eventful and productive life. Even at a young age, he went through a number of changes in the direction of his education, beginning at Manual Training High School in Brooklyn, which taught students to build things with their own hands. Later in his research career, he thought that this training enabled him to design and build the specialized equipment he needed, but upon graduation he quickly started looking in other directions. He entertained ideas of going into either electrical engineering or vaudeville (it was the 1920s) but eventually rejected both and took up law studies at the Washington Square College of New York University. Law didn't hold his attention for long either, though; in his own words, he wanted something "more substantial, more natural, more organic" (36). He enrolled in premedical education but lost interest in medicine before committing too much time to it. Then he got the idea that biological research might be worth pursuing. He applied for graduate studies in zoology at Columbia University, was accepted, and began the research trajectory that saw him win a share of the Nobel Prize in Physiology or Medicine in 1967. From the time he began research on vision, as a graduate student, to the end of his life, Wald also progressed through a number of issues that interested or concerned him, aside from his first research love, vision.

When he arrived at Columbia as a new graduate student, Wald met the famous fruit fly geneticist Thomas Hunt Morgan, who would have impressed him, as he had so many other smart people, with his brilliant development of genetics. But the person who had a greater direct effect on him was Selig Hecht, who would become his research mentor and point him in the direction of his life's research. Hecht was a biologist interested in vision who had been profoundly influenced by the emerging idea that physics and chemistry should be used to describe biological phenomena. He planted this idea in his students' heads. In his view, biology should progress from largely observational research to include the language of quantitation and chemical structure. This turned out to be both prescient on his part and useful for his new student Wald, who would later acknowledge that Hecht had a profound effect on both his research orientation and his general approach to science and life — he had been a mentor in many respects.

After completing his PhD in 1932, Wald travelled to Europe to spend a "wander year" in three famous laboratories, where he hoped to learn more about vision and to develop his research expertise generally. The first place he visited was the laboratory of Otto Warburg, one of a formidable group of scientists who commanded the biochemical research world of Germany. There were hints and clues that vitamin A was involved in vision, and in Warburg's laboratory, Wald thought he had identified vitamin A in the retina of the eye. He next worked in the laboratory of Paul Karrer, in Switzerland. Karrer was the chemist who had determined the structure of vitamin A and beta-carotene. Wald wanted to use his time there to confirm that what he had found in the eye while working in Warburg's lab was indeed vitamin A, and in just a short time, he did. But although vitamin A was present in parts of the eye, its function there, and whether it was directly involved in vision, had yet to be settled. In 1933, in another German laboratory, Wald brought his European tour to an end because of the growing political discomfort for Jews in that country (Wald was Jewish). Before he left, as a final push deeper into vision research, he found that there were two different forms of vitamin A in the retinas of frogs, and that their interconversion was caused by light (see Figure 5). This was a profoundly important clue to how vision works, and it set him on a productive research path.

At that point, Wald, still in his 20s, returned to the United States and the University of Chicago. A year later he got a job as an instructor at Harvard University. He was to remain there for the rest of his academic career, rising in rank as he excelled in both research and teaching.

Each summer, Wald would travel to the Marine Biological Laboratory at Woods Hole, in Maine, where he studied the visual pigments in the rods of marine animals and taught students enrolled in a summer research course. He discovered that different species of fish had slightly different visual pigments, but all of the pigments contained vitamin A. Later it became clear that the differences between rhodopsin, the sensitive visual pigment that provides night vision, and the cone cell "conopsins," the visual pigments for colour vision in brighter light, were due to their different protein components. The visual chromophores, the coloured small molecules bound to the visual pigment proteins, were the same aldehyde forms of vitamin A, retinal. A key finding about the role of retinal in vision was uncovered by Wald's second wife, Ruth Hubbard, who showed that retinol and retinal could be interconverted.

George Wald's academic activities were not limited to research. He was also a gifted and dedicated teacher, "one of Harvard's best" (36). In 1960 he began teaching an introductory biology course called "The Nature of Living Things," which he taught for the rest of his life (he died in 1997). The two semesters of the course were initiated by lectures titled, respectively, "Origin of Life" and "Origin of Death," and they covered, among other subjects, cosmology, atoms, molecules, and all aspects of biology. The related laboratory manual gained national attention, and at one point *Time* magazine named him one of the country's 10 best teachers. Beginning around the time of the war in Vietnam, he also became more interested in politics, devoting himself to subjects such as opposition to that war, stopping the proliferation of nuclear arms, and limiting the expansion of the military–industrial complex.

In 1986 Wald and a number of other Nobel Prize winners were invited to Moscow to advise Mikhail Gorbachev, leader of the Soviet Union, on environmental questions. He used the opportunity to ask Gorbachev about the internal exile of the Soviet physicist Andrei Sakharov; "internal exile" meant that the person was forced to live in a remote Siberian city and forbidden to live and work in Moscow. Sakharov had designed the Soviet Union's thermonuclear weapon (a hydrogen bomb) but subsequently became concerned about the implications of his work and began

to campaign for civil liberties and reform, and against nuclear proliferation. For this activity, he won the Nobel Peace Prize in 1975. But after he
publicly protested against the Soviet invasion of Afghanistan, he was "rewarded" with internal exile in 1980. Gorbachev claimed to know nothing
about what had happened to Sakharov, but shortly after Wald's visit, the
scientist was released from exile and allowed to return to Moscow with his
wife. George Wald's was a wide ranging, productive, and interesting life,
in keeping with the characteristics he showed as a youth.

In the famous 1958 paper, Wald and Harvard undergraduate John
Dowling described, step by step, what happens during vitamin A deficiency in the rat. From what we know today, it closely reflects the results
observed in vitamin A-deficient humans. In that publication (37), Dowling and Wald carefully described the timing of events that followed the
removal of vitamin A from the diets of male albino rats. They measured
the levels of vitamin A in the bodies of the rats, as well as the state of the
rhodopsin in their eyes, at various times. The visual acuity of the animals
was determined by anaesthetising them and determining how much light
was required to elicit an electrical response in the visual system to the
brain. With these tools, the investigators looked at the whole picture of
what vitamin A deficiency meant, over time.

They knew already that the liver in rats, as in humans and other
mammals, is a reservoir of vitamin A in a well-fed individual and can for
a time provide a buffer when the vitamin is missing from the diet. This
is in contrast to the water-soluble vitamins, which need to be replaced
on an almost daily basis. In the rats of Dowling and Wald's study, the
only change over the first four weeks (Figure 6) was that the liver levels
of vitamin A declined almost to zero over about three weeks. The moment that happened, blood vitamin A plummeted, as the blood is not a
reservoir — it is just a means for distributing the vitamin from the liver
to the tissues that need it. The next change was in rhodopsin, the visual
pigment; as vitamin A levels fell, rhodopsin lost its retinal component and
vision deteriorated. Finally, opsin, the protein component of rhodopsin,
also began to disappear.

Without a supply of vitamin A, the rhodopsin levels in the rod cells of the eye began to decline after four weeks. By five weeks they were down by 20%, and by six weeks, 40%. As rhodopsin declined, so did vision, as detected electrophysiologically: the brains of the rats were receiving weaker signals, ones that corresponded to nightblindness in humans. Notably, the loss of vision was more dramatic than the loss of rhodopsin; a 20% drop in rhodopsin at five weeks led to a more than 10-fold loss of vision. As rhodopsin levels declined because of a loss of retinal, its protein component, opsin, also began to disappear. By eight weeks, the visual acuity of the rats was down to one-thousandth of the initial values.

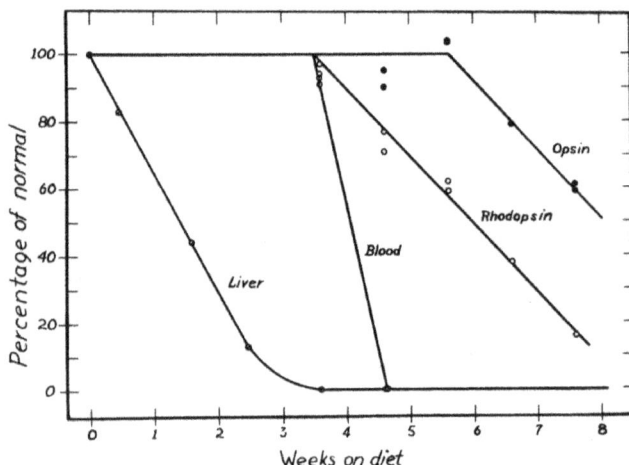

Figure 6. *The effects of vitamin A deficiency on rats. Albino rats were deprived of vitamin A. This resulted in a decline in their liver vitamin A levels, followed by a loss of blood vitamin A and of rhodopsin in their eyes. As rhodopsin dwindled, opsin, its protein component, also began to decline. (Taken from (37), with permission.)*

Between six and eight weeks, something new happened: there was catastrophic damage to the epithelial tissue of the eye and other organs, and by eight weeks, most of the rats were dead. What was the connection, if any, between the death of the rats and the loss of vision? Microscopic examination showed that the loss of vitamin A during the first six weeks, although it led to a decline in vision, had little effect on the integrity of the epithelial tissue — the histology was normal. But by eight weeks, there were profound changes in the pigment epithelium, the tissue that overlays the rods and cones.

While the loss of vitamin A (as retinal) led to a progressive loss of rhodopsin, it was the deterioration of epithelial tissue throughout the body — reflected by what was happening in the eye — that led to death. As Dowling and Wald commented, the only function of vitamin A that was clearly understood in 1958 was supplying the visual chromophore of the eye, "[which] plays only a trivial role in the whole complex of vitamin A deficiency. No animal dies of nightblindness."

Vitamin A regulates genes essential for life

The two kinds of results seen by Wald and Dowling — blindness and death — were due to the loss of two different forms of vitamin A. Retinal, the aldehyde version, is the visual chromophore, which captures light and initiates an activation signal to the brain. But the damage to epithelial tisue that they saw at later stages, which led to the deaths of the rats, were due to a lack of retinoic acid. This was made evident by their further work, carried out when Dowling had become a graduate student. It showed that retinoic acid prevented the devastating effects of vitamin A deficiency, including death (38), but it didn't cure blindness, because it cannot be converted back to retinal or retinol (Figure 4). They made explicit what became the basis for our modern understanding: that retinal is involved in vision, but the functions essential for life found by them and earlier by others were served by retinoic acid.

Today we understand many of the physical and chemical steps that link the absorption of a photon by retinal to subsequent events in the visual process (Figure 5). Although the details of those steps are complex, the overall pathway is not as complicated as the role of retinoic acid in gene regulation, which is responsible for the more pervasive health effects of vitamin A. It has been known for almost a hundred years that a vitamin A deficiency in laboratory animals has profound effects on all aspects of their health. If the deficiency is severe, reproduction stops; we now know that maturation of reproductive organs requires vitamin A (39).

The specialized functions of many highly differentiated tissues require vitamin A — specifically, retinoic acid — including tissues involved in the immune response, bone growth, reproduction, the surface linings of the eyes, and the epithelial integrity of the respiratory, urinary, and intestinal tracts and the genitalia (40). More properties are being discovered every year; there are, on average, two new peer-reviewed publications a day about vitamin A, almost all of them concerned with the functions of retinoic acid. Indeed, despite the effects of a deficiency of retinal on the eye, by far the most devastating effects of vitamin A deficiency are due to a lack of retinoic acid, which led to the deaths of albino rats as originally seen in 1913 but soon also observed in guinea pigs, dogs, rabbits, and humans (41). The unexpected deaths of vitamin A-deficient children in Indonesia, noticed by Alfred Sommer, were undoubtedly the result of a loss of retinoic acid. And the effects of retinoic acid deficiency can be traced to a failure in gene regulation in specialized tissue.

The events of the 1980s saw a dramatic change in how scientists and physicians regarded vitamin A. The beginning of the turnaround was the observation by Sommer and others of the untimely deaths of vitamin A-deprived children in Indonesia, an event already outlined in the first chapter and considered in more detail in the chapter on vitamin A's effects on human health. Then, in 1987, shortly after the initial clinical trials of vitamin A had taken place in several developing countries, there was a discovery that would eventually explain the essential life-sustaining properties of vitamin A: two groups of scientists, one in France and the other in the United States, found that the nuclei of many kinds of cells contained proteins that bind retinoic acid (Figure 3) (42, 43). These nuclear proteins, when activated by binding retinoic acid, attach to regulatory sequences of genes (regions of DNA outside the protein-coding parts) that control how strongly a gene will be expressed. Genes regulated by vitamin A are inactive and unexpressed in the absence of the activating proteins with their bound retinoic acid; once the complex of retinoic acid and its receptor protein binds to the regulatory region of DNA, the affected gene can be expressed. Retinoic acid activates a genetic switch.

The proteins that bind retinoic acid in the nuclei of cells, called retinoic acid receptors (RARs), were discovered in 1987. They were soon found to be somewhat related in structure to known receptors for steroid hormones, thyroid hormones, and vitamin D, each of which regulates the expression of different genes. But the story of RARs rapidly became much more complex than that of any of those other gene activators, as the number of RARs increased to three, with each a product of a separate gene. The multiplicity did not end there; it turned out that the products of each of the RAR genes were processed into different forms, with slightly altered properties. Then, an obligatory second protein, a "facilitating factor," was discovered, which was required for the effective functioning of the RAR–retinoic acid complex. This second family of gene-activating proteins was called RXRs, and here too there were three major gene products, and various altered forms (44). The RARs and RXRs associated pairwise in different combinations, increasing the number of options for their effects. It was further discovered that another, completely different, nuclear regulatory protein could also bind retinoic acid (44).

In addition to being a gene-activating trigger on its own, the retinoic acid gene-signalling pathway is connected to the paths of the thyroid hormone receptor and the vitamin D receptors, which affect the expression of other genes. Furthermore, the retinoic acid system can also alter the response to signals delivered by agents such as peptide hormones. In another twist, the retinoic acid nuclear receptor appears to block some gene expression when retinoic acid is not present (45), so it can be an "off-switch" as well as an on-switch. One of the discoverers of the retinoic acid receptors, Pierre Chambon, from Strasbourg, France, asserted in 1996 that the complexity of retinoic acid signalling "has no counterpart in other vertebrate nuclear receptor signalling systems (e.g., steroid hormones)" (44).

Retinoic acid regulates the expression of more than 500 genes (46). Some of these are involved in the highly differentiated functions of cells and tissues, including the maintenance of normal epithelial structure and function — the loss of which was responsible for the deaths of vitamin A-deprived rats observed by Dowling and Wald. Its importance can be seen in the immune system, which consists of highly differentiated cells and molecules that prevent damage from invading entities such as viruses, bacteria, and toxins. Many forms of immune response are diminished by vitamin A deficiency (47-49), increasing susceptibility to infection. The immune system is also regulated to prevent over-reaction, such as occurs in hypersensitivity to certain allergens or in autoimmunity. The prevention of autoimmunity is dependent on retinoic acid, acting on different genes from those required for the immune response (50). These regulatory effects of retinoic acid on the immune system are the results of complex patterns of retinoic acid-related gene expression, mediated by the RAR–RXR system.

Given this complexity of effects, how do we categorize vitamin A? Some authors refer to it as "hormone-like"; some even call it a "hormone." But it isn't a hormone, like insulin or adrenaline. Those substances are produced by endocrine glands in response to the body's changing needs. In the case of insulin, there are glucose receptors on pancreatic beta cells. As blood glucose levels rise, these cells initiate increased insulin production and secretion into the blood; the insulin then causes a number of tissues to take up glucose and either use it for energy production or convert it to fat for energy storage. In the case of adrenaline, the adrenal medulla is the responding gland. As a result of a neural signal that indicates a need for a strong physical reaction, the adrenal medulla secretes adrenaline into the blood, and adrenaline increases the capacity of muscle and other cells to "fight or flee."

But retinoic acid isn't like that; it must be present at all times to maintain certain cellular activities. How a cell uses retinoic acid in its day-to-day life is determined by the cell's particular interior environment. This includes the kinds of gene products that a highly differentiated cell contains, such as particular gene-regulatory proteins and cell-surface receptors. If, for example, a cell is genetically programmed to reduce an inappropriate autoimmune response, it will need to express the appropriate RAR and RXR factors (as well as other gene-regulatory proteins) so that it can carry out that predetermined function.

Another aspect of retinoic acid's complexity is that it can work on genes directly to turn them on (or sometimes off), or it can activate genes that produce secondary genetic regulatory factors (46). In this indirect mode of action, retinoic acid (bound to the proper RAR–RXR complex) binds to the control region of a particular gene, switching on the production of its protein product, and this protein product in turn switches on a second gene. Retinoic acid–RAR–RXR switch molecules can also be modulated by other cellular events to have greater or lesser activity, depending on what else is going on in the cell (51). The complexity of its gene regulatory pathways is at the heart of the complexity of vitamin A.

One of the roles of vitamin A is to help orchestrate embryogenesis. For example, in the developing mouse embryo, retinoic acid increases the expression of a particular developmentally critical gene in one part of the embryo while suppressing it in another (52). This is essential for the creation of a viable embryo, with its head-to-toe spectrum of differences. As in other examples, vitamin A is not a specific trigger for development, but it is a necessary factor for development to occur. Its known effects on a galaxy of genes help explain the observations that in laboratory animals, maternal vitamin A deficiency can result in placental dysfunction, stillbirths, developmental problems, and congenital malformations (39, 47, 53-56).

Some plants contain provitamin A

The beta-carotene found in plants (Figure 2) has several important properties. The chemist's eye sees a system of conjugated double bonds (illustrated for retinol in Figure 1), which creates an electron-sharing environment, with "delocalized" electrons buzzing around in it. There is a relationship between the size of a delocalized system (the number of conjugated double bonds involved) and the light energy it can absorb: The larger the system, the longer the wavelength of light it is activated by, and the lower the energy of that light. Beta-carotene absorbs blue light (which makes it appear yellow-orange), and it contributes some of this energy to photosynthesis (35). Its absorption spectrum thereby complements that of chlorophyll in extracting energy from sunlight. Beta-carotene consists of two basic units of vitamin A, joined by a double bond that is also conjugated with those of its vitamin A units. This means that the conjugated double-bond system in beta-carotene has 11 double bonds, many more than retinol, which has only five. As a result, beta-carotene absorbs (longer wavelength, lower energy) visible light, while free retinol absorbs in the ultraviolet (higher-energy) part of the spectrum.[15] The conjugated double-bond system of beta-carotene also creates an efficient "sink" for free radicals (molecules with unpaired electrons). This means it is an antioxidant that can neutralize reactive oxygen species, which are responsible for tissue damage to lipids, proteins, and DNA (34, 57).

Plants such as the orange sweet potato have the genes required for the synthesis of beta-carotene in their leaves. So, they are in the genome and potentially available for its production in the root tuber as well. Sweet potatoes were presumably subject to a variety of growing conditions through their evolution. Quite possibly, sweet potatoes growing in some habitats are well served by having the antioxidant beta-carotene present in their below-ground tubers. There are also purple sweet potatoes, whose colour is due to another class of antioxidants, the anthocyanins. Red beets derive their colour from yet another antioxidant, betanin. A number of other food plants also contain antioxidants in their roots, including the mango and liquorice. Perhaps all of these antioxidants are protections against certain soil conditions or damaging agents. Whatever the biological advantages of their beta-carotenes, the orange sweet potato is now being used to meet human needs for vitamin A in parts of Africa, as we will examine in Chapter 5.

Vitamin A has a long and broad involvement in life on earth. It is present as light-sensitive retinal-protein structures in all three kingdoms of life: bacteria, archae,[16] and eukaryotes (cells with nuclei). Some bacteria have rhodopsin in their outer membranes, using it to collect light

---

15 11-cis retinal, with six double bonds, and bound to opsin in an energetic, torqued conformation in the retina of the eye, does absorb visible light. Being bound to the protein opsin accounts for the difference from free retinal.

16 The archae, formerly known as archaebacteria, look like bacteria and, like bacteria, have no cell nucleus, but they are evolutionarily closer to eukaryotes (organisms with nucleated cells) than to true bacteria.

energy and to pump out sodium ions (58). Archae use bacteriorhodopsin to generate energy directly or to pump ions across their membranes (59). The eukaryotes, including plants, animals, and everything else with a cell nucleus, use it for the purposes already described, including vision and photosynthesis.

Archae are ancestrally related to the eukaryotes, including humans. It might be logical to assume that their opsin protein is evolutionarily related to the opsin in human eyes, but it isn't. The rhodopsin of archae contains retinal, and its protein component consists of seven coiled helixes that wind back and forth across the membrane of the cell. Both features are also characteristic of mammalian opsin. But genetic analysis tells us that the opsin proteins of archae and the eukaryotes evolved separately (59, 60). What drove the evolution of the two opsin forms was the usefulness of the available chromophore retinal, which they bind and utilize. Biologists refer to such evolution as "convergent," where different structures evolve to a common or similar function.

Regarding the other class of vitamin A functions — the regulation of gene expression — the retinoic acid-binding nuclear proteins involved in that process represent yet another, separate, evolutionary development that is unique to eukaryotic cells.

The list of functions for carotenoids such as beta-carotene is long and varied. To that list, one reviewer has added: "to attract pollinators, to advertise ripe fruits as a meal in exchange for seed dispersal, to maintain ranks in schools of fish, to attract a mate, to provide camouflage" (61). The carotenoids have a history of versatility.

CHAPTER 4

Vitamin A and Human Health

We have known about the effects of vitamin A on human health for much longer than we have understood what vitamin A is. One of the earliest references to the effects of vitamin A on vision is contained in a document known as the "Ebers Papyrus," which is in the library of the University of Leipzig, in Germany. It is thought to date from about 1550 BCE, and it represents the state of medical knowledge in Egypt at that time. Among the subjects it addresses is nightblindness, the loss of vision in low light, for which the recommended cure was pressing roasted ox liver to the eye. Although there can be other causes for this condition, vitamin A deficiency is the most common one, and liver is a rich source of the vitamin; consuming liver remains an effective treatment. In more recent times, nutritional scientists discovered that diets containing adequate protein, carbohydrate, fat, and salts, but not the right kind of micronutrients, failed to sustain the lives of laboratory animals. This led them to the discovery, and rediscovery, of the "other nutrients" essential for life. One of these was "fat-soluble A," renamed vitamin A, which is present in milk fat and other foods, as described by McCollum in 1913 (8).

In addition to the risk of scurvy due to a lack of vitamin C, many sailors in earlier times also experienced nightblindness on long voyages — after a few weeks away from land, some would lose the ability to see in dim light. This nightblindness was caused by a deficiency of vitamin A in their diets, just as it was for the Indonesian children being studied by Alfred Sommer in the late 1970s. Some sailors developed more serious eye problems, including "dry eye syndrome," which is a further stage of deterioration caused by vitamin A deficiency. This condition is part of xerophthalmia, a process of deterioration of the eye's cornea and conjunctiva. In later stages of xerophthalmia, the eye becomes ulcerated, keratinized, and covered with insoluble protein plaques, a condition known as keratomalacia. This is followed by total blindness and, if the deficiency persists, death.

In the early 19th century, the French physiologist Magendie noticed that malnourished laboratory dogs, in addition to having an increased death rate, suffered from corneal ulcers. The malnourishment consisted of feeding the dogs almost entirely only sugar water. His physician colleague Charles Billard thought he saw a connection between what happened to Magendie's dogs and to some malnourished children. There was, at the time, a steady inflow of abandoned infants in Paris. These were babies who had been born to poor women, many from outside the city, and brought to Paris so that they could be "found." Professional "baby-finders" roamed the city, picking up abandoned infants and taking them to a Catholic "foundling hospital," where the finder was paid by the nuns. (The nuns, in turn, received operating funds from the city in proportion to the number of foundlings in their care.) Billard, working at one of the foundling hospitals, noticed that the symptoms of many of these infants resembled those of Magendie's malnourished dogs (62). In addition to losing their vision, many of the infants died of infectious diseases. Today, we recognize that both of these outcomes can result from vitamin A deficiency. In terms of the effects described in the previous chapter, the first of these is caused by a deficiency of retinol, the second by a lack of retinoic acid.

How World War I led to vitamin A deficiency in Denmark

Some of the clearest evidence that a fat-soluble substance present in dairy products was required for human health was observed in Denmark in the years bracketing World War I, and that evidence was a direct result of the war. Before 1912, serious xerophthalmia, involving deterioration of the cornea and conjunctiva of the eye, was rare in Denmark, as it was in most European countries. There were reports of keratomalacia, one of the late stages of xerophthalmia, from around the world, and their common feature was poor nutrition, either of the sufferer or of the mother around the time of the sufferer's birth. But it was seldom seen in the Scandinavian countries. Then, inexplicably, the number of cases of xerophthalmia in Danish children began to increase rapidly, although in other Scandinavian countries, such as Sweden, it stayed low. Each year between 1911 and 1917, that number went up, as documented by the Danish paediatrician Carl Edvard Bloch, who described the course of the outbreak in children in Copenhagen during those years (63). Bloch noticed that before they suffered the effects on their eyes, the children first lost weight and generally failed to thrive — he described them as "miserably emaciated." Very few adults were afflicted by these symptoms.

When Bloch first published his observations on the Danish children, he was not aware of the concurrent work of the American nutritional scientists, McCollum and the others, who defined "fat-soluble A" in 1913. But he did know of the work of the Japanese physician Masamichi Mori. Between 1896 and 1904, Mori had studied a group of 1,500 children under the age of four who lived in a mountainous area of Japan and whose diets lacked milk, fish, and fat in general (64). Many of these children suffered from a condition called "Hikan," known in Japan since ancient times. Their symptoms included nightblindness, diarrhoea, corneal ulcers, total blindness, and increased mortality. The symptoms of Hikan were those that we attribute to vitamin A deficiency. Hikan was found almost exclusively in children living in poor circumstances inland, whose diet contained little fat, but seldom in children who lived near the sea, whose diet included fish. Mori felt that a lack of dietary fat was at the root of the disease. The notion that a missing component of the diet could cause a disease ran counter to the prevailing paradigm, which was that diseases are caused by infectious agents, as indeed the work of Pasteur, Lister, Koch, and others had shown.

As had Mori, Bloch treated his patients, the Danish children, with cod liver oil and whole milk, and those who were not too seriously ill recovered. But those in the latter stages of xerophthalmia, such as keratomalacia, often did not. He thought that their disease was related to the lack of certain "lipoid bodies," present in particular kinds of fat. He differed in his thinking from Mori, who attributed the effects on the Japanese children to an overall lack of dietary fat. The affected Danish children had fat in their diets, but it was lard, animal fat that didn't contain an essential micronutrient, which Bloch felt could only be provided by certain fats. Then he became aware of the work of McCollum and other nutritional scientists on "fat-soluble A." Without this dietary component, the rats studied by McCollum failed to grow, suffered visual impairment, and died. Bloch saw a parallel between his young patients in Copenhagen and the rats suffering vitamin A deficiency in a laboratory in the American Midwest, including the ability of milk and cod liver oil to cure the condition.

In 1917, during the course of his observations, Bloch came upon some cases originating in a children's home (an orphanage) in whose administration he was involved. In particular, the cases of xerophthalmia came from only one of the four sections of the home, and they all arose over a period of a few months. The symptoms of the affected children included eye problems and weight loss. Bloch found that all children were being given sufficient quantities of protein, fat, carbohydrate, and salts. But the affected children had had essentially no whole milk, only partially skimmed milk, for many months, while the healthy children had received whole milk daily. The affected children were treated with cod liver oil, and their symptoms diminished. They were subsequently given whole milk as a normal part of their diet. Bloch also noted that vegetable margarine did not replace dairy in providing the essential "fat-soluble A."

Returning to the troublesome larger picture, of increasing levels of xerophthalmia in the Copenhagen hospital, Bloch noted that nearly all cases came from rural areas, from the poorest and most destitute homes, the households of labourers, herdsmen, and the "poorest cottagers." The milk that these children did receive was skimmed; the butterfat went to dairies to produce butter, much of it for export to remedy Denmark's finances. These children were eating margarine, made from imported vegetable oil, which Bloch already knew did not replace dairy as a source of "fat-soluble A." He also noted that the disease was almost always seen in rapidly growing children, who, he reasoned, required more of the missing "fat-soluble A." Bloch in essence had mapped the results of the American scientists' work on rats onto the health of Danish children.

There was a sudden change in the number of cases of xerophthalmia in Copenhagen in 1918; it dropped to just one. The explanation wasn't that children were suddenly being treated at outlying hospitals. The answer lay in outside events: in February 1917, Germany established a submarine blockade around Denmark, which stopped the import of plant oil used for margarine production and of cattle feed. As the feed became scarcer, milk production decreased a little, and pig production (the source of the lard being given to poor children) almost stopped. The blockade also halted the export of butter, so butter consumption within Denmark actually increased. This caused a steep rise in the price of butter, and more and more of Denmark's poor could not afford it, so on December 21, 1917, butter rationing began, with every person being entitled to 250 grams a week at a controlled price affordable for even the poorest residents. The cases of xerophthalmia in Copenhagen fell to near zero the next year.

A fuller explanation of what happened came from a comprehensive study carried out by another Danish physician, Olaf Blegvad, and published in 1924 (65). Blegvad was appointed by the Ophthalmological Society of Copenhagen to examine keratomalacia in children throughout Denmark.[17] As mentioned earlier, in keratomalacia, there is extensive ulceration of the cornea. It is a very serious condition and can quickly be followed by complete blindness and death. Blegvad looked at data obtained throughout the country and over a longer span of years, and he also examined the level of butter production and the importation of plant oil for margarine production. As in Bloch's report, almost all of the victims of keratomalacia were children of poor parents. The therapy was to give them whole milk and/or cod liver oil, but even with this treatment, the outcome — in contrast to the recovery from some of the milder forms of

---

17 Blegvad and Bloch used the terms "xerophthalmia" and "keratomalacia" somewhat interchangeably. They were undoubtedly looking mostly at serious cases of vitamin A deficiency, so keratomalacia is probably a correct term for all of those outcomes. Blegvad actually did include a small number of less severe cases of xerophthalmia in his overall investigation, but he kept these separate from the keratomalacia cases.

xerophthalmia — was grim: death occurred in 22% of cases, and of the survivors, 27% were completely blind, 24% had very poor vision in both eyes, and 35% had poor vision in one eye. Blegvad's data provided a more thorough test of Bloch's theory that xerophthalmia was due to a dietary lack of a crucial fat-soluble nutrient (vitamin A). It showed a close temporal relationship between cases of keratomalacia and the importation of vegetable oil for margarine production (Figure 1). As oil imports increased and butter consumption by poor people dwindled, the number of cases rose; when the German submarine blockade was established in 1917, the importing of plant oil and the number of cases of keratomalacia dropped precipitously. But after the blockade was lifted at the end of the war, in 1918, plant oil imports increased again, and the number of cases of keratomalacia also began to increase.

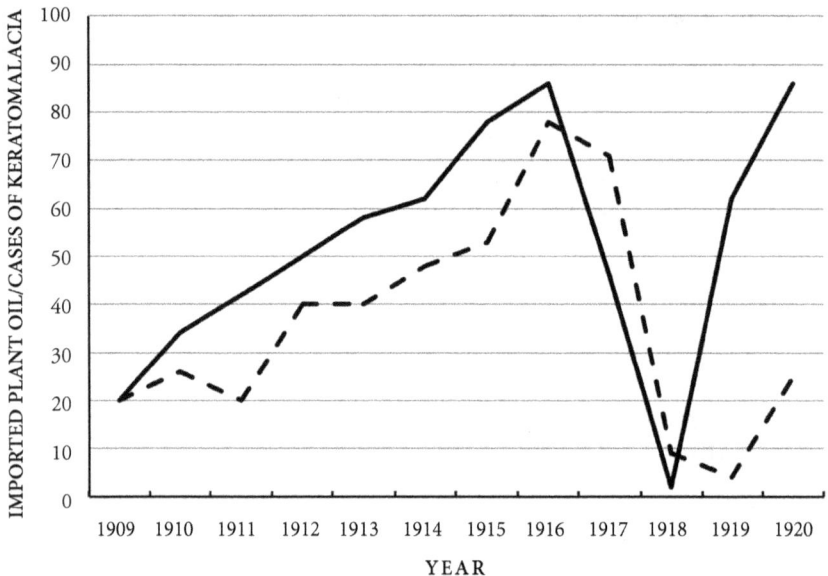

Figure 1. *Correlation between cases of keratomalacia in children in Denmark (broken line) and the relative level of consumption of plant oil used to produce margarine as a replacement for butter (solid line). After oil used for margarine production was cut off by a submarine blockade, the number of cases of keratomalacia fell, but note the upward trend after 1919. Data from Blegvad (65).*

Bloch's description of the xerophthalmia outbreak and its causes was originally published in Danish and wasn't noticed by the rest of the world until being republished, in English, in 1921 (63). He had noticed that the reduction in margarine production was a result of the German blockade, and that it led to an increase in butter consumption by poor people. In a subsequent note attached to the English translation of his work, he predicted that the incidence of xerophthalmia would again rise after the end of the war, as price controls on butter were removed and poor people began to eat margarine again. And Blegvad's data do in fact show a small increase after 1918 (Figure 1).

Blegvad also realized a more subtle point: that it wasn't enough to have vitamin A in the diet — if the diet was poor in fat, the vitamin would not be taken up during digestion. Given the predominance of the disease in children, he agreed with Bloch's conclusion that growing children "used up" vitamin A more rapidly than adults did and would suffer sooner from its absence. This phenomenon is seen in poor societies experiencing vitamin A deficiency today, where it is principally the children who suffer. We also know that the uptake of vitamin A or of beta-carotene is reduced if the overall fat content of the diet is too low. Blegvad noted that keratomalacia was occurring in some very young children, most of whom were still nursing, and often it was the mothers who had a deficiency of vitamin A and therefore were unable to pass it on to their babies. Clearly, the substitution of margarine for butter among the poorest people in Denmark was the cause of keratomalacia, not a decrease in butter production; butter production actually declined a little in 1917 due to the German blockade, yet the cases of keratomalacia dropped, within months, to near zero.

Vitamin A, the "anti-infective" agent

The Danish experience, and also that of Mori in Japan, showed that milk and cod liver oil contain a nutrient that is important in the human diet. A direct indication that supplemental vitamin A could improve health in some situations was uncovered by the English physician and scientist George Mellanby in the early decades of the 20th century. Mellanby, a former student of Hopkins, was carrying forward Hopkins' work on essential nutrients, using dogs and rats in laboratory experiments. At the time, vitamin A was defined as the fat-soluble trace nutrient in liver and dairy; it could be destroyed by a heating protocol developed by Hopkins, which allowed Mellanby to distinguish the effects of vitamins A and D (66, 67). At one point, a group of dogs being bred by Mellanby for nutritional studies, some of which were on vitamin A-deficient diets, developed bronchopneumonia. Mellanby noticed that the pneumonia was confined to the vitamin A-deficient dogs, and further experiments showed that this relationship also held for rats — a diet lacking in vitamin A made the animals susceptible to infection (66).

Based on his animal experiments, Mellanby wondered whether it would be beneficial to give his human patients supplemental vitamin A, as a way of reducing their chances of getting an infectious disease. He addressed this question in collaboration with his colleague Dr. H. N. Green. Following a small but encouraging preliminary study, Mellanby and Green set up a larger one on pregnant women entering Jessop Hospital in Sheffield, England, to deliver their babies. An important health risk following childbirth was "childbed fever," due to puerperal sepsis. Puerperal sepsis is caused by infection of a newly delivered mother's reproductive tract with one of several common bacteria, and it was an ever-present, mortal danger before antibiotics. Mellanby wondered whether he might be able to help women avoid serious puerperal sepsis following childbirth by giving them a vitamin A supplement. He provided part of a group of pregnant women with vitamin A for several months before they entered hospital, and compared their health after delivering their babies with the health of women who hadn't received the supplement. The results, published in 1931, were striking (68). Vitamin A reduced the incidence of serious puerperal sepsis from 4.7% to 1.1%, a reduction of 77%. Although the women in Mellanby's test group stopped taking vitamin A before they went into the hospital for delivery, that didn't matter, because the vitamin stored in the liver provides protection for several months. The dramatic reduction in puerperal fever was related to the need of pregnant women and new mothers for a higher level of vitamin A than usual, because they are passing the vitamin on to their babies in utero before birth, and through their breast milk afterwards. The women's vitamin A needs to ensure their general well-being and their ability to resist infection were not being met by their normal diets. As a result of his studies, Mellanby coined the phrase "anti-infective agent" for vitamin A.

Although Mellanby's insight into the role of vitamin A in preventing infection was an important advance, like so many parts of the story of vitamin A, it was not the first time such observations had been made. A different Japanese scientist named Mori (not Masamichi, of the Hikan experience) had seen that in vitamin A-deficient rats there was atrophy of mucus-secreting cells in several tissues, and that these tissues became sites of bacterial infection (69). Mellanby was aware of Mori's work, and he put his own efforts with his patients in the context of what the Japanese investigator had seen with rats.

A further confirmation of the importance of vitamin A for health took place soon after Mellanby's studies, again in England. Before there was a vaccine, measles was a recurring nightmare, with bad outbreaks almost every other year in that country. Hospital wards would be over-flowing with measles patients, and before the 20th century, up to 20% of children who entered hospital with measles in England died. An assistant medical officer with the London Fever Hospital, Joseph Ellison, was aware of the work of both Mellanby and Mori (the one who worked with rats). He thought that children with measles might be helped by giving them cod liver oil (which contains vitamin A). The death rate of the treated children was about half that of the other children, as he reported in 1932 (70). Again, it seemed clear that vitamin A had an "anti-infective" power, in the sense that it limited the measles infection. It was an observation that cried out for further investigation.

Vitamin A was also being studied for effects on tissue, aside from its role as an "anti-infective agent." These studies concluded that it was essential for maintaining the function and integrity of epithelial tissue, which lines the body's cavities and organs, including the surfaces of blood vessels. Vitamin A deficiency resulted in epithelial cells becom-ing keratinized, losing their moisture and becoming hard and horn-like

(41). The tissue around the eyes became encrusted, tissue of the respiratory tract deteriorated, and there were dysfunctional changes to the digestive tract as well as the reproductive organs, thymus, spleen, and lymph glands. These changes did not require infection — they were apparently direct effects on the epithelial cells themselves. This showed that vitamin A had a more complex impact than just blocking infections, a theme that continued to develop over the following decades. These effects are consistent with the known science of vitamin A, which has shown that maintenance of differentiated tissue function, such as the characteristic structure of epithelial cells, depends on gene-regulatory events in the nuclei of the cells involved.

By 1940, at least 30 studies — the majority of them in the United States — had been conducted to see whether vitamin A could reduce infections and mortality (5). But the results were mixed; some studies showed that vitamin A had efficacy, some didn't. In part, this was because general health conditions, including nutrition, had improved in most of the modern world, and vitamin A deficiency was becoming less common. If a patient already had a satisfactory level of vitamin A, there would be no further beneficial effect, in terms of disease prevention, of giving a supplement (a principle to keep in mind in today's world of ubiquitous vitamin supplements). Reflecting the improved living conditions in the more developed nations, the infant mortality rate (i.e., death within the first year of life) in the United States fell from about 25% in 1920 to 4.8% in 1940. Part of this overall improvement resulted from the use of cod liver oil as a daily supplement for the child. The same improved conditions were probably also responsible for a continuing decrease in the death rate from measles. As conditions of hygiene and diet improved, the overall death rates from infectious diseases decreased. Even during Ellison's time, death rates from confirmed cases of measles in England were dropping (5), although it remained a continuing problem until a vaccine became available in 1963. But probably the most important development in the medical landscape, one that effectively ended the interest in vitamin A as an "anti-infective agent," was the discovery of antibiotics. Beginning with the sulpha drugs in the 1930s, and continuing with the miracle of penicillin in the early 1940s, the medical world felt that it now had "magic bullets" that could cure any bacterial infection. In Europe and North America, which is where essentially all of the research on the effects of vitamin A was going on, there was no longer a need for "extra" vitamin A, above what was contained in a good mixed diet.

The role of vitamin A in vision was given molecular definition by the work of Dowling and Wald in the late 1950s. But as antibiotics and immunization came to the fore, the experiences of earlier medical researchers, such as Mellanby and Ellison, with vitamin A as a disease-preventative mechanism were largely — but not completely — forgotten. A reminder that vitamin A deficiency has an impact on global health issues, including infectious diseases, was provided by reports to the WHO in 1962 and 1968 (71), in which its role was comprehensively reviewed. The 1968 report summarized the importance of nutrition for infection and concluded that "[v]itamin A deficiency shows synergism with almost every known infectious disease." In other words, whatever else is contributing to a disease condition, vitamin A deficiency often plays a role. The WHO report showed that this applies to many human diseases and to a wide array of animal ones as well, including infectious diseases caused by bacteria, viruses, and protozoa[18]. Based on those reports, it was unwise to disregard the role of vitamin A in human disease. Subsequent events confirmed that conclusion and showed again how important vitamin A is in maintaining overall health and resistance to infectious disease.

Vitamin A, anti-infective agent redux

Vitamin A's essential role in human life asserted itself again in the early 1980s, beginning with the epidemiological study carried out by the group of investigators from Johns Hopkins University led by Alfred Sommer, as described in Chapter 1. This time, its effects were seen in rural Indonesia, where diets were less well rounded than in the developed world. Sommer travelled to Indonesia in 1977 to study nightblindness in children living in

---

18 Protozoa are single-celled animals that live in the body and cause disease; malaria and sleeping sickness are caused by protozoa.

rural areas of that country. He, his wife, and their two young children arrived in the city of Bandung, 140 kilometres southeast of Jakarta, where Eijkman, Pekelharing, and their Dutch colleagues had first identified vitamin B1 (thiamin) 90 years earlier. Sommer was there to study vision loss due to vitamin A deficiency. This could be most easily investigated in a population that was known to have a relatively high level of nightblindness, as was the case in the rural area that had been the target of the first study. As epidemiologists interested in unusual diseases well know, and as Sommer said in his popular account of that time, you must "[g]o where the problems are" (1) to understand them — in other words, go to a place where the incidence of the problem is high. Vision loss due to vitamin A deficiency had almost completely disappeared in more developed parts of the world due to improved nutrition, but it was ubiquitous in rural Indonesia.

Sommer's group set up several studies related to vitamin A deficiency and visual problems. One of them was centred in a hospital to which children suffering the more severe effects of xerophthalmia were being brought. Soon after his arrival, Sommer saw a young patient with a serious case of xerophthalmia. The boy was in danger of going blind, and Sommer needed to treat his condition immediately (72). But a technical problem — the solubility of vitamin A — made the obvious treatment challenging. Earlier in his career Sommer had been part of an advisory group helping the WHO create protocols for treating vitamin A deficiency. Vitamin A doesn't dissolve in water; it was originally called "fat-soluble A" for that reason. Vitamin A deficiency was being treated by injecting it under the skin in an oil base. This turned out to be largely useless; the oily drop just sat there, a lump under the skin, and didn't significantly increase the level of circulating vitamin A. The WHO decided, as a result of the meeting of the advisory group in which Sommer participated, that a water-soluble form of the vitamin should be used as the injectable treatment. So when faced with the case of serious xerophthalmia in rural Indonesia, Sommer asked the hospital authorities for water-soluble, injectable vitamin A. The puzzled officials informed him that it didn't exist, not in the hospital, not in Indonesia, not anywhere. Even though it had been recommended by the WHO as the best way to treat acute vitamin A deficiency, it had never been produced by any pharmaceutical company. Sommer was faced with treating the child using the only available form of vitamin A, the oil-based formulation, which he knew was almost useless when injected. So he improvised: he loaded a syringe with the oil-based vitamin preparation and squirted it into the boy's mouth, in hopes that it would be absorbed in the gut. And that worked very well. The child's vitamin A levels increased, and his symptoms and vision improved. Sommer had used a form of the vitamin that was essentially like that available to the people living in fishing villages in Scotland, Sweden, and Norway in the 19th century. He had administered a kind of synthetic cod liver oil orally. Nevertheless, he immediately contacted the pharmaceutical company Roche and told them to get busy and provide a water-based form of vitamin A.

The water-soluble form turned out not to be needed, as the oral route for oil-based vitamin A preparations worked well. This was fortunate, from a logistical and financial point of view, since the vitamin was easily given even by a non-medical person (injection required medical expertise), and the cost was about two cents a dose (whereas the water-soluble vitamin preparation was much more expensive). The hospital-based study of the progression of xerophthalmia, from mild (symptoms of nightblindness and Bitot's spots[19] to severe (complete destruction of the epithelium of the cornea and blindness), and the ability of vitamin A to reverse it, could now be started.

But it was the field study, which was separate from the hospital-based work, that provided the surprising result when Sommer was re-examining the data during that fateful Christmas week in 1982. In that study, the children were being examined at three-month intervals for both general health and visual problems. It was known that the vast majority of cases of xerophthalmia were preschool-age children, so that was the group being studied. And as described in Chapter 1, the surprising result was that children who had experienced even the mildest symptoms of xerophthalmia,

---

19 Bitot's spots are an early indication of vitamin A deficiency. They consist of raised, foamy or pearly-appearing patches on the conjunctiva of the eye, due to deposits of an insoluble protein called keratin.

nightblindness, which had often spontaneously reversed, were at greater risk of dying than those who hadn't. And the worse their symptoms, the more likely they were to die subsequently. Severe forms of xerophthalmia, such as the keratomalacia observed by Blegvad in Norway, were associated with a high likelihood of death, sometimes approaching 100% (64, 73). What was new, and shocking, was that by the time a child showed signs of nightblindness, which was considered to be a relatively benign condition that could easily be treated or that would spontaneously reverse, that child was already in mortal danger. If the study's results were right, nightblindness was an advanced stage of overall damage due to vitamin A deficiency. Sommer published that surprising result in the high-profile medical journal *The Lancet* (74). In Sommer's own words, it was "greeted with less than a yawn" (1), and it went almost completely unremarked and unnoticed. It was clear that the medical establishment was not ready to understand and accept its implications. Those who may have read the publication presumably thought its conclusions must be wrong; the problem couldn't be that simple.

By the time Sommer realized what the first study had implied about nightblindness and childhood deaths, the Johns Hopkins group had organized another study in Indonesia, which was about to begin. It was designed to look for beneficial effects of vitamin A on vision in even larger groups of children. The initial aim of the second study was to see whether children given vitamin A prophylactically would have better eye health. To try to answer the question raised by the earlier results — i.e., whether vitamin A might affect mortality — Sommer quickly added another question to the design of the second clinical trial: What was the mortality of children given vitamin A every six months, compared to those who received nothing? Some 26,000 children in 450 villages in Aceh province, in northern Sumatra, were randomly assigned to either a treatment group (200,000 international units of vitamin A administered twice over a period of a year) or a control group (who received no supplements). All of the children were given vitamin A after the end of the study.

In well-controlled clinical trials, the subjects are separated, randomly, into a treatment group and a control group, and neither they nor the trial doctors know who is in which group until the study ends. This is called a "double-blind" study. The control group is given a placebo that physically resembles the treatment agent. This wasn't possible in the vitamin A trial, but there was a solution that was almost as good. The government of Indonesia wanted to eventually provide all children with vitamin A, but because of the scope of the government program, it had to be introduced in five parts, starting at different times. Initially, children in some areas would be given vitamin A, while others would not yet receive the vitamin. The researchers asked to have villages assigned to the treatment group randomly. So there were children, in randomly selected villages, who had not been treated, and they therefore provided the control data. The "double-blind" approach wasn't possible, but there was a reason subjectivity or bias wasn't thought to be a significant problem: death is a "hard endpoint," in the jargon of epidemiology, and is not subject to interpretation.

Over a one-year period, providing vitamin A every six months reduced xerophthalmia by 75% for children up to 71 months of age, as expected. The effect on mortality was even more dramatic than expected from the earlier study, and the results were also published in *The Lancet*, in 1986 (75): death from all causes was reduced by 34% in children receiving vitamin A prophylactically. In these communities, young children often died of measles, bronchopneumonia, or diarrhoea, and vitamin A supplementation, just as for Mellanby's and Ellison's study populations 50 and 60 years earlier, reduced deaths from infectious diseases. The paradigm of vitamin A as the "anti-infective agent" had been forgotten by the medical establishment; neither of the *Lancet* papers published by Sommer and his collaborators in 1983 and 1986 referenced it. He has since remarked that he had been unaware of those earlier results and the way that vitamin A had been viewed decades earlier.

The second *Lancet* paper, in contrast to the first, generated a strong reaction within the international medical community. It was difficult to accept that vitamin A could dramatically reduce death from all causes among preschool children. Yet what had been demonstrated, more convincingly than previously, was consistent with what Ellison and Mellanby had observed — vitamin A could reduce deaths from infectious diseases in children who were vitamin A deficient to begin with. The Indonesian children, like the ones whom Ellison had seen 50 years earlier, were often vitamin A deficient, contracted infectious diseases at a high rate, and frequently died from them. If Ellison's conclusions were acceptable, then why not those of the team studying vitamin A supplements in Indonesia?

Confirming the essential role of vitamin A was a challenge

A single study of this type, complex in structure and fraught with difficulties in execution, could not by itself prove the point, radical in the eyes of the medical community, that vitamin A has lifesaving properties. Follow-up studies were required, and this effort was already underway. An even larger study was being organized in the Philippines, but this one met catastrophe. In his definitive treatise on vitamin A, Richard D. Semba describes in detail what happened (13). The study was to take place in the Albay province of the Bicol region in the Philippines, beginning in 1986, and was also being organized by the Johns Hopkins team. The field director was Kate Burns, a nurse with several years' experience in public health in Africa. Hundreds of local applicants for fieldworker jobs were interviewed, and thousands of homes were visited to enrol some 40,000 children. A pilot study went well. The team was poised to begin.

But the timing of the project was unfortunate. Earlier in 1986, the president of the Philippines, Ferdinand Marcos, had just completed his 20th year in office. Marcos had risen to power with the strong backing of the United States, which wanted to maintain its air force base in the country. Marcos ran the Philippines with an iron hand and for his own financial benefit. In 1972, he declared martial law, and he continued to control the country as a dictator until 1981. He was subsequently re-elected as President, and the Congress was re-established, but all of his electoral victories were questionable. It was said that Marcos had stolen millions of dollars from his country and squirreled them away in private Swiss bank accounts, but that turned out to be incorrect — the amount stolen was billions, not millions. In 1983, his political opponent, Benigno Aquino, Jr., returning from medical treatment in the United States, was taken off his plane at Manila International Airport and assassinated; the general opinion was that Marcos' supporters were responsible.

Marcos called a snap election on February 7, 1986 to reaffirm his control of the country and reduce criticism of him. The campaign was marked by violence and vote tampering by his supporters. According to his own campaign officials, Marcos won. According to independent poll watchers, the winner was Aquino's widow, Corazon. An instantaneous and peaceful uprising blocked Marcos' inauguration. He turned to his traditional ally, the United States, but that avenue had been closed off; President Reagan, finally seeing more realistically what was going on in the Philippines, turned away from him. The American ambassador, Stephen Bosworth, delivered the message from Reagan to Marcos: Reagan, it said in part, looked forward to Mr. Marcos "working out a scenario for a transition government" and would welcome him and his family if they wanted to move to the United States. Nine days after the election, Marcos and his shoe-loving wife, Imelda, boarded a United States military helicopter and left for exile in Hawaii, and Corazon Aquino became the President of the Philippines.

The vitamin A study was to begin that summer. To quote Semba on what happened next (13):

> [O]n Thursday morning, August 21, 1986, the residents of Bicol awakened to unwelcome news: Nelson Arao, a popular radio announcer, told his listeners that more than two dozen children in Albay had fallen ill with nausea, vomiting, and diarrhoea after being given a vitamin A capsule. The source of the news . . . was Frances Burgos, a young Philippine physician who headed the Bicol chapter of the Medical Action Group, which had been founded in response to perceived human rights violations during the Marcos administration. This group had an anti-American slant because of the previous support that America had provided for Marcos. Arao then broadcast a Medical Action Group statement that American researchers were using the children of Albay province "as guinea pigs." (page 172)

Ever more hysterical uproar followed, including charges that the United States was dumping unwanted vitamin A capsules in the Philippines, and that it was doing this to stimulate future demand for them. The term "international conspiracy" was heard. Dr. Burgos brought children ostensibly poisoned by vitamin A to a regional health office. Allegations of death caused by vitamin A surfaced. All of the objections were based on unsubstantiated claims, but it didn't matter. The opposition grew to include members of the New People's Army (the regular armed forces of the Communist Party of the Philippines), who threatened fieldworkers. Mothers began to withdraw their children from the study, and some questioned the safety of childhood immunization programs against tetanus, diphtheria, and whooping cough, asking whether the vaccines also contained vitamin A.

By this time, Marcos was gone, his departure having been negotiated by the Americans. But the anti-American sentiment established earlier was a formidable force, and the American-led clinical research project on Filipino children was vigorously opposed by many groups in that country. The Johns Hopkins researchers knew when they were beaten; they packed up their equipment, closed the offices, and moved the study to Nepal. The vocally anti-American Dr. Burgos, apparently able to master his previous revulsion for America, subsequently left to take up medical practice in Phoenix, Arizona. Dr. Sommer commented that he couldn't think of anything the Johns Hopkins group could have done differently to overcome the resistance. The New People's Army marched on to oppose a number of other projects in the Bicol region, including a World Bank initiative to manage community resources. Twenty-seven years later, it was instrumental in blocking an attempt to test a new method of overcoming vitamin A deficiency by using genetically modified rice, as will be described in Chapter 6. In the meantime, it oppressed the population, killing many citizens and abusing the civil rights of even more.

Although the effort in the Philippines to reproduce the results of the Indonesian study could not be carried out, other studies were more successful. This included the one in Nepal organized by the Johns Hopkins group.

Clinical trials in the developing world, especially those involving large numbers of people, are difficult and can fail for a number of reasons. The Bicol study failed for ideological reasons. Another study in Khartoum, Sudan, which was started in 1988, also failed, this time because of a natural disaster. A massive flood of the Nile river caused a disruption of the study population, and as the emergency was ending, local officials gave all children vitamin A supplements, negating any conclusions that might have been drawn. Nevertheless, the coterie of those opposing vitamin A supplementation, about which more will be said, often refers to the failed Khartoum study as demonstrating a lack of effect on childhood mortality. It didn't. It was compromised by circumstances and the behaviour of local officials and proved nothing.

On top of the difficulties provided by the particular conditions of studies in developing countries, clinical studies like these are inherently demanding. They are expensive, and the required organizational support is complex. They need to be well led and clearly conceived, with well-thought-out objectives and end points. And they need to be sensitive to local conditions and customs, and accepted by the community.

Given the potential for failure, the study in Nepal achieved impressive results, which showed that vitamin A supplementation reduced death from all causes in the population of young children (i.e., six to 60 months old) by 30% (76). Boys and girls were equally affected. The study was prospective, randomized, double-blind, and placebo-controlled, and it included enough subjects (28,630 children) to enable statistically valid conclusions. Being prospective rather than retrospective, it directly asked: What will be the future effect of this particular treatment on this particular outcome? Randomization ensured that pre-existing differences between the children in the treated and control group were averaged out. Double-blind meant that neither the subjects nor the staff knew who was in which group, and so they could not, consciously or unconsciously, bias the data. A clinical trial structured with these features is referred to as adhering to the "gold standard"; it answers virtually all possible objections that can be raised as to its reliability and conclusions.

As a further test of the ability of vitamin A supplements to have an effect on mortality, the control group of children in the Nepalese study were given vitamin A after the study ended at 12 months and then were observed further. Between 16 and 24 months after the study had been started — that is, between four and 12 months after they had been given vitamin A supplements — their relative risk of dying was essentially the same as that of the children who had been getting vitamin A supplements all along. In other words, vitamin A reduces the risk of dying almost immediately. It clearly can reverse pre-existing conditions that threaten the health of children (77).

Another study, in Ghana (78), saw mortality from all causes decrease by 19% through vitamin A supplementation; morbidity (in this case, the severity of diarrhoea experienced by the children) was also reduced significantly. As evidence of the effectiveness of vitamin A supplements, while reports of home illness in that study were the same for the control and supplemented groups, the frequency of hospital visits was reduced by 38% for the treated group, reflecting a reduction in the number of more serious illnesses.

Vitamin A deficiency in the world

The early studies, and others that were well controlled and constructed, showed that vitamin A supplementation in developing countries reduces childhood deaths from all causes. It was also evident that the risk of death exists even when there aren't signs of visual impairment (79). This was consistent with studies from the 1930s, which showed that changes to epithelial structures preceded involvement of the eyes (41). Countries that have attained a high level of coverage with vitamin A supplements have seen the virtual disappearance of hospital admissions of children with nightblindness and other symptoms of xerophthalmia. Among preschool children, xerophthalmia can be reduced 60–90% by the simple expedient of providing a large dose of vitamin A every six months (see page 184 of (80)).

In a complex issue such as the effect of vitamin A deficiency on health, a form of statistical analysis called "meta-analysis" is often used. In meta-analysis, all of the relevant studies are combined to extract the most accurate overall conclusion. A meta-analysis can be as simple as just taking all the relevant results and combining them, giving each study a weight proportional to the number of subjects included in it. More sophisticated statistical methods can also be used, such as giving weight to a study in proportion to its quality — how well it was controlled, for example. A meta-analysis seeks patterns of outcomes and consensus conclusions, and it highlights areas of agreement and disagreement between studies.

A meta-analysis carried out at the University of Toronto in 1993 on all available studies concluded that childhood mortality in developing countries was reduced by 23% by vitamin A supplementation (81). Another such study, at Harvard, indicated that the number was 30% (82). An analysis done at Oxford University, combining the best studies carried out up to 2011, showed a 24% reduction in childhood mortality when children were provided with high-dose vitamin A capsules, and the researchers concluded that worldwide, 600,000 children were dying of vitamin A deficiency each year (83).

Vitamin A supplementation in the diets of reproductive-age women in Nepal reduced pregnancy-related deaths by 40%, as documented in a study published in 1999 (84). An analysis of available data in 2004 predicted the number of children and pregnant women dying prematurely as a result of vitamin A deficiency, worldwide, was about 800,000 (85). Another analysis, in 2008, indicated 350,000 (86). It has been estimated that in India alone, two million children under the age of five are dying each year (13). Given the documented vitamin A deficiency in India, the number of children dying because of vitamin A deficiency could be around 500,000 annually in that country alone. Another estimate, in 2012, put the total number of children's deaths that could be prevented by vitamin A supplementation world-wide at 1.9 to 2.7 million a year (87). It is not surprising that there are various answers to the question of how many childhood deaths are due to vitamin A deficiency. Human health is incredibly complex and is subject to different variables in different parts of the world. And in the analyses themselves, studies may be weighted for perceived quality, or they may include additional data if done at another time. But by anyone's analysis, any of these numbers is far too large.

Most studies on vitamin A have concluded that the benefits of vitamin A supplementation in children are seen most acutely between the ages of six and 72 months, and that there is little effect on infants younger than six months old (88). This may be because pre- and post-natally, babies derive vitamin A from their mothers. This improves the odds of the infant surviving the first six months of life but increases the risk that the mother will contract a serious illness if her diet is deficient in vitamin A. As already indicated, pregnant women and nursing mothers are also a population at risk of vitamin A deficiency. For them, the result is usually nightblindness (89).

The WHO has tried to estimate how many children are affected worldwide and what should be done. It's a difficult task. For one thing, vitamin A deficiency is often a concomitant of deficiencies in other essential micronutrients, including minerals and other vitamins, and such additional deficiencies will contribute to health outcomes. Globally, the most common micronutrient deficiency is iron, which affects the oxygen-carrying capacity of the blood, the effectiveness of the immune system, and the functions of hormones (90). The effects of different micronutrient deficiencies on each other are often difficult to tease out; a deficiency in one, such as zinc, may have an impact on the requirements for another, such as vitamin A. Also, conditions in various countries change constantly. Such changing conditions may include better (or worse) nutrition, resulting in lesser (or greater) health risks, or immunization programs that prevent diseases such as, for example, measles. While it is impossible to derive a precise figure for the number of people seriously affected by a deficiency of vitamin A, it is unquestionably large. That number is changing, going down in many countries where programs are in place to provide vitamin A supplements. But clearly, clinical trials have shown that supplementing vitamin A in young children and pregnant women saves lives.

The WHO has tried to estimate the effects of vitamin A deficiency and in 2013 concluded that of the 190–250 million people worldwide who are vitamin A deficient, there are some 250,000–500,000 children who go blind each year, and about half of these die (89). By that estimate, 125,000–250,000 children a year are dying of vitamin A deficiency. The

WHO estimated that in 2015, a total of around six million children died from all causes in South and Southeast Asia, sub-Saharan Africa, and parts of Central America. That number is going down, slowly, as a result of better nutrition and hygiene, and of immunization programs. If, as seems plausible from the analyses of all existing studies, 25% of these children could be saved by vitamin A supplementation, the number of children dying of vitamin A deficiency could be as high as 1.5 million a year — much higher than the official WHO estimate. Children in some of these countries are already beneficiaries of vitamin A supplementation, as will be described in the following chapter, so 1.5 million is probably an upper limit. But experts with direct experience of children with vitamin A deficiency provide higher numbers than the WHO.

How do these results relate to what is known about the science of vitamin A? Clearly, human nightblindness is similar to the early stages of vision loss seen by Dowling and Wald in their vitamin A-deficient rats in 1958 (37). It is caused by the loss of retinal in the rhodopsin molecular complex in the retina when blood retinol levels fall, leading to a loss of vision in dim light. But other serious outcomes of vitamin A deficiency arise from deep-seated cellular effects, which reflect the multiple gene-regulatory activities of retinoic acid. These result in the degradation of epithelial cells, as has been known about for almost 100 years (41). In the case of the eye, the symptoms begin with the "dry-eye" syndrome, which was noted for, among others, sailors on long voyages hundreds of years ago (the Greeks were also aware of "dry-eye syndrome"; xerophthalmia is their word). Dowling and Wald also documented that retinoic acid prevented the more serious tissue damage to the eye characterizing the later stages of xerophthalmia; however, because retinoic acid cannot be converted back to retinal, the visual pigment, it could not prevent the progressive blindness in their rats (38). When there is sufficient retinol (or its ester forms), there will also be a supply of retinal and retinoic acid, since retinol is converted to these forms.

The deaths of children deficient in vitamin A can also be caused by the inability of the immune system to prevent infections, which can lead to serious illness, including dehydration due to diarrhoea. This again reflects the fitness of Mellanby's "anti-infective agent" label for vitamin A (91). The mechanism by which vitamin A affects the immune response is similar to its effects on epithelial cells: retinol is converted to retinoic acid, which combines with specific proteins in the nucleus of the cell to form gene-regulatory factors. The genes affected are critical for the immune response to disease agents such as viruses and bacteria. The structure and function of epithelial cells throughout the body are also part of vitamin A's protective effect against infection. Epithelial cells form the lining of the digestive tract and other surfaces and are a barrier to infection. When epithelial cells are damaged or not functional due to vitamin A deficiency, infectious agents have an easier entry route.

Facts and myths about high levels of vitamins

Most vitamins have few toxic effects when taken in excess of their RDA (recommended daily allowance). But excess vitamin D, which is a fat-soluble vitamin, like vitamin A, causes a rise in blood calcium levels, resulting in loss of appetite and feelings of nausea. Simply reducing the intake of vitamin D relieves the symptoms. It is quite difficult to get an excess of vitamin D from a normal diet or exposure to sunlight, and vitamin D toxicity is so rare that it isn't even clear what levels are unsafe. Because some recent evidence suggests that higher vitamin D levels may be linked to reduced risk of illnesses such as cardiovascular disease and cancer, the RDA could go up in the future. But even at its present value, it has been claimed that some 42% of Americans are deficient in their blood vitamin D levels (92) (there are differences of opinion about that number). Like vitamin A, vitamin D is present in the liver, and cod liver oil was a source of the "sunshine vitamin" in winter-dark places for over a hundred years.

Proponents of the idea that consumption of large amounts of vitamin C (ascorbic acid) could solve a plethora of medical problems, including the common cold, cancer, and schizophrenia, have recommended that people take hundreds of milligrams of it a day (the RDA is between 50 and 100 milligrams). This elevated intake level was first proposed by one of the most famous chemists of the 20th century, Linus Pauling (he won two Nobel Prizes, one for Chemistry and one for Peace), and is still a subject of intense debate for some people. However, existing scientific evidence of the kind published in peer-reviewed research journals provides no clear evidence for a beneficial effect in terms of curing cancer (93) or schizophrenia (94). For certain groups of people, megadoses of vitamin C, if taken all the time, may reduce the risk of getting a cold, or the length of time that cold symptoms persist, but there is not much of an effect if it's taken after the cold starts (95). Periodically, there are fresh claims of benefits from hypervitaminosis C, but so far, these claims have not stood up to further scrutiny. Vitamin C is not known to be dangerous, but excess consumption can lead to painful urination, kidney stones, and the enrichment of vitamin supplement companies.

Another of the water-soluble B vitamins, niacin (vitamin B3), has a curious history of overdosing related to illegal drug use. Niacin has the reputation of enhancing the rate of drug metabolism and masking illegal substances in urine tests, and some users have taken massive doses for this purpose. In one case (96), a 14-year-old boy on probation had smoked a lot of marijuana and, in the 36 hours before meeting his parole officer, took a huge dose of niacin, almost a thousand times the RDA. On the day of the meeting, he felt dizzy getting out of bed. Despite taking such a massive overdose, his symptoms quickly disappeared when he stopped taking the vitamin (there's no record of the results of his meeting with his parole officer). No amount of niacin-containing food can produce such levels of this vitamin; only over-the-counter supplements can do that. The water-soluble B vitamins like thiamin do not stay in the body long — they are rapidly absorbed in the gut, travel to the muscles and to organs such as the liver to do their respective jobs, and are then eliminated from the body.

A deficiency of Vitamin A is life-threatening — it is an essential dietary micronutrient for humans. But in contrast to many other vitamins, an overdose of vitamin A can be toxic, and this must be kept in mind when devising supplementation or fortification schemes. Excess vitamin A causes blurred vision, dizziness, vomiting, anorexia, headaches, and any number of more permanent effects if the overdosing continues. Dietary vitamin A that is in excess of immediate needs is stored, with the liver normally containing 90% of the body's supply. The liver's ability to store large quantities of vitamin A is both an advantage and a potential problem. The advantage is that humans can survive by receiving a single huge dose of vitamin A every few months. Even a relatively large dose of vitamin A can be safely stored in the liver and then released if there isn't much of it in the diet during the intervening time. That's why programs that provide supplemental vitamin A to children in need are effective, as was seen in the studies carried out by the Johns Hopkins teams in Indonesia, which gave a relatively massive dose of preformed vitamin A every four to six months. But it is better to provide a continuous source of vitamin A, either preformed (as retinol or its esters) or in provitamin form (via plants containing beta-carotene) in the regular diet. Mechanisms for achieving that through the fortification of foods are available, as I will describe in later chapters.

Toxicity due to extreme vitamin A dosage has occasionally been seen. Eating animal liver that contains excessively high levels of vitamin A is the most usual cause. Animals living in the Arctic are efficient at storing vitamin A, and their livers may contain so much vitamin A that they are acutely toxic to humans eating them. Consuming the livers of polar bears is particularly dangerous. On a Danish expedition to East Greenland in 1913, a polar bear was killed and a stew made of its liver, heart, and kidneys (97). According to the record of the expedition's doctor, Jens Peter Johannes Lindhard, two to four hours after the meal, symptoms began to appear. These included drowsiness, sluggishness, irritability, or an irresistible desire to sleep, as well as severe headaches and vomiting. On the second day, the skin of 10 of the 19 men affected began to peel around the mouth, gradually spreading over larger areas. In several cases the skin peeling became quite general. When this report, and similar ones describing unfortunate encounters between explorers and the livers of certain arctic animals, were analyzed in 1943, it became clear that vitamin A toxicity was undoubtedly responsible for the symptoms (97). Polar bear liver contains some 30 to 60 times more vitamin A per gram than the liver of a well-fed human, and halibut liver is even higher (98). The skin peeling observed in a number of the victims is characteristic of retinoids used to reduce acne and other skin conditions (which I will describe below) (99). We now know that the chronic intake of excess vitamin A can lead to increased intracranial pressure, dizziness, nausea, headaches, skin irritation, pain in the joints and bones, coma, and even death.

Circumstantial evidence for the toxic effects of elevated vitamin A on human health may go back a long way. The remains of early hominids found at Lake Turkana, in Kenya, by the anthropologist Richard Leakey and his colleagues show a symptom consistent with chronic excess vitamin A ingestion — osteoporosis (100). These skeletons date from about 1.5 million years ago. The researchers attributed this disorder to a high intake of carnivore liver in the diet, at a time when dietary practices were changing to include hunted animals, and before it was learned by experience that it's best not to eat some parts of some animals.

Dosage must be taken into account when considering the toxic and beneficial effects of vitamin A. The amount of preformed vitamin A can be measured as either the weight of pure retinol, the basic dietary form of vitamin A, or as International Units (IU); one IU is defined as 0.3 micrograms of the pure chemical. (One IU of beta-carotene is 0.6 micrograms of the provitamin.) The RDA for preformed vitamin A in North America is 3,000 IU per day for adult men and 2,300 for women; an acutely toxic dose — the amount of retinol that would immediately cause toxic effects — is estimated to be about 25,000 IU per kilogram of body weight. For a 25 kg child, this corresponds to 600,000 IU, which is (only) three times higher than the dose administered in supplementation studies in the developing world (usually 200,000 IU every four to six months).

Perhaps the most contentious question of toxicity pertaining to hypervitaminosis A (i.e., overdose) is whether it is teratogenic — that is, if a pregnant woman consumes high levels of vitamin A, will her child have birth defects? This question was thrust into the public consciousness by a paper published in *The New England Journal of Medicine* in 1995 (101). The authors claimed that women who took in more than 10,000 IU of vitamin A daily had a significantly higher chance of delivering a baby with malformation of parts of the brain, spinal cord, or heart ("cranial-neural-crest"). That research was featured in an article in *The New York Times* and has been referred to frequently by both proponents and critics of its conclusions. The most worrisome finding was that for women who daily consumed more than 10,000 IU of preformed vitamin A as supplements, the risk of these types of birth defects more than quadrupled.

This study illustrates some of the difficulties with studying human nutrition. A number of experts wrote critical letters to *The New England Journal of Medicine* in the following months. They pointed out the small size of the effect being described. Almost 23,000 pregnancies were included in the study, of which 339 babies showed evidence of birth defects. Of those, 121 were judged to be of the "cranial-neural-crest" type, and in this group were nine babies born to mothers who recalled that they took more than 10,000 IU of vitamin A a day. Statistically, there should only have been two to three, so the conclusion was based on six or seven babies out of 23,000 delivered. The critics raised other points. They questioned the categorizations of the birth defects, which were done by the obstetrician or the mother, stating that they should have been carried out, or at least confirmed, by an expert in the area. One critic also pointed out that some important data were not in the paper, and that this omission may have compromised the conclusions.[20] Finally, some critics expressed a concern that the prominent reporting of this study in the popular media might have the effect of causing pregnant women to avoid taking recommended multivitamin supplements during their pregnancies.

In any case, subsequent research has strongly questioned the proposed linkage between moderately high vitamin A intake and birth defects. An investigation published in 1997 directly contradicted the 1995 paper (102). A review of existing information in a study organized by the WHO also concluded that 10,000 IU per day was safe during pregnancy, and that even a much higher level of vitamin A intake by women did not

---

20 Many medical science reports, such as this 1995 study, consist of showing a correlation between two variables and implying that one caused the other. Yet there may be other variables affecting the outcomes in a given set of circumstances, and both events may have been caused by another event altogether. Correlation does not equal causation. For example, in the USA between 1998 and 2007, there is an almost perfect correlation between expenditures on organic food by consumers and reported cases of autism. And there is a very good correlation between the amount of chocolate consumed by each citizen of a country and its number of Nobel Prize winners per 10 million people.

present a risk (103). Since it would be unethical to expose pregnant women to very high levels of vitamin A, given the possibility that it causes birth defects, a clever approach was used by another group to study the effects of increased levels of vitamin A (104). Non-pregnant women were given high levels of vitamin A, up to 30,000 IU per day, for three weeks. Their serum levels of retinoic acid (which was presumed to be the substance causing the birth defects) were found to be essentially the same as those of pregnant women on "healthful" levels of the vitamin, and these levels were known not to cause birth defects in primates.

It is true that hypervitaminosis A causes birth defects in laboratory animals, but the amounts required are more than 100 times the RDA for those animals (105). This has no bearing on pregnant women taking amounts of vitamin A around two to three times the RDA. Again, it is worth remembering that forms of provitamin A such as beta-carotene, which is found in certain foods, have never been shown to cause birth defects in laboratory animals, and such sources of the vitamin are undoubtedly safe for humans in almost any amount. (That said, if your skin turns orange, it is probably wise to cut back, if only for cosmetic reasons.)

Although the linkage of preformed vitamin A to birth defects is questionable, there is a serious risk attached to the use of a compound called isotretinoin, formerly commercially available as Accutane.[21] This acne medication is known to cause birth defects in primates (106). Some human babies born to mothers taking Accutane did indeed have birth defects. The pharmaceutical company Roche, the inventors of the drug, took it off the market in 2009, by which time the patent had expired and generic versions were available. It remains on the market today, although its use is heavily regulated, as any pregnant woman in the Western world will probably know. It presumably causes birth defects in primates because it closely resembles retinoic acid, and the body can convert it into that substance. It also resembles chemically altered versions of retinoic acid that can damage a developing embryo.

---

21 Isotretinoin is retinoic acid that has undergone a rotation around one of its double bonds. We call such substances "isomers"; they have the same chemical formula but different chemical structures, and this difference can affect how they interact with other substances.

Another pregnancy-related condition in which there may be a linkage to vitamin A metabolism is fetal alcohol spectrum disorder (FASD) (107). FASD is a nutritional disease resulting from excess alcohol consumption by a pregnant woman. In addition to other effects, alcohol may interfere with vitamin A metabolism and thereby cause birth defects (108). Ethanol (the intoxicating substance in alcoholic beverages) affects vitamin A distribution in the body and competes for the enzymes that convert retinol to retinoic acid (109); this conversion to retinoic acid is critical in the early stages of embryo development (110). There is further support for the notion that at least part of the developmental damage caused by ethanol is due to its effects on vitamin A pathways. In rodents administered ethanol during pregnancy (to model the conditions leading to FASD), the ethanol inhibits the activation of retinoic acid receptors (111); conversely, ethanol-caused birth defects are prevented by retinoic acid (112). It may be that ethanol interferes with the production and actions of retinoic acid.

Giving high doses of vitamin A to children deficient in the vitamin is beneficial, but well-fed children may have adverse (although not life-threatening) episodes. In Ecuador, vitamin A supplementation reduced the incidence of lower respiratory infection in undernourished children, but for children of normal weight — which suggested they had better nutrition — it actually increased the frequency and severity of such infection. In neither the undernourished children nor the children of normal weight was the risk of death increased (113). These and other studies support the notion that while undernourished children are often helped by supplementary vitamin A, those who have an adequate level of vitamin A in their bodies may experience short-term illness. It would be better for everyone to have a continuous daily source of either preformed vitamin A or provitamin A, but this is not yet possible.

Another factor that may affect the response to administered vitamin A is a difference in sensitivity due to genetics. There is evidence that in at least one case of acute dietary vitamin A overdose (children in a family were being given far too much vitamin A), siblings differed significantly in their susceptibility to being overloaded with the vitamin (114). This adds to the number of factors that influence the response to vitamin A, and it further argues for the idea that a moderate, continuous source of the vitamin is preferable to receiving a large dose infrequently.

The balance between potential life-saving effects (decreased mortality) and increased non-life-threatening effects (increased morbidity) is not uncommon for any type of public health intervention. Among preschool children receiving the large, semi-annual dosages of vitamin A typically used in developing world countries, five to 10 percent may experience one or more short-term, limited symptoms, including nausea, vomiting, headache, and/or fever. Such symptoms usually last no more than 24–48 hours (115, 116).

In one case in India, the presumption of vitamin A's toxicity has had a profound effect on supplementation programs. This situation illustrates how complex and misguided public health policy becomes when poor science, nationalistic pride, and confusion are in play (117). As will be described in a subsequent chapter, international efforts to prevent blindness and death due to vitamin A deficiency in children have given rise to supplementation programs in developing nations. One of these efforts was directed at the children of Assam, in northeastern India, in 2001. Under the aegis of the WHO and with the agreement of the Indian national government, a one-day "pulse" of oral vitamin A delivery was carried out in conjunction with the administration of oral polio vaccine the same day.[22] Children throughout the province were given 200,000 IU of liquid vitamin A, the dosage recommended by WHO. However, there was soon a rising level of criticism, primarily from a small group of Indian paediatricians and nutritional experts who claimed that the intervention had resulted in 14 deaths and thousands of illnesses among the treated children over the following week (118). Accusations of fraud and greed were levelled, along with claims that the project was driven by the pharmaceutical industry, which wanted to gain a future market for their vitamin A products. These criticisms and accusations were reminiscent of the outcry that had stopped the clinical trial of vitamin A supplementation in the Philippines in 1984. But the claim of excess deaths was statistically

---

22 Experience in India has shown that such one-day "pulse" campaigns are the most efficient way to achieve wide coverage.

meaningless (119). That day, 2.5 million children had been treated. In that place and at that time, the death rate for children was around seven per thousand per year; the number of children's deaths in an average week would therefore have been about 350 amongst those 2.5 million. The 14 deaths to which critics pointed provided no evidence that the vitamin A supplements had caused them. As for the thousands of illnesses, it is true that a certain percentage of children receiving a vitamin A supplement develop nausea, headaches, and diarrhoea, but these symptoms disappear in a day or two. Nevertheless, this "scandal" led some influential Indian authorities to resist supplementation, and the effects of their opposition persist to this day.

As well as the toxicity associated with a single, massive overdose of vitamin A, chronic intake of vitamin A levels that are higher than the RDA is correlated with increases in osteoporosis and hip fracture in older people. This observed association is consistent with data showing that lower bone density results from excess vitamin A. A Swedish study found that an increased retinol intake for 20 years by men initially aged 49–51 was correlated with an increased likelihood of bone fractures of any kind; similar results have been obtained in the United States. The threshold level for such effects was just 5,000 IU per day, which was associated with a doubled risk of fracture (120). Such an effect would be consistent with observations from laboratory studies showing that vitamin A affects bone remodelling, increasing the rate of bone resorption and decreasing the rate of bone formation (121). This may be related to the effect of vitamin A on vitamin D function (vitamin D normally increases bone density). The Swedish bone-fracture data suggest that a toxic effect is observed at less than twice the recommended daily intake. In view of this, it is worrisome that vitamin A supplements contain from 4,000 to as much as 25,000 IU of preformed vitamin A per dose. (Pills containing 10,000 IU are commonly available from health food stores, pharmacies, and online vendors, including Amazon.)

Before 2001, the RDA set by the Food and Nutrition Board of the US Institute of Medicine was 5,000 IU per day for men, and the "tolerable upper intake level" for preformed vitamin A was 10,000 IU per day (the exact dosage that many popular vitamin A supplements claim to provide). That RDA is presumably the basis for the relatively high dosages of vitamin A supplements. Today's RDAs for men and women in the United States are 3,000 and 2,300 IU per day, respectively. For children aged one to eight years, the RDA is about 1,000 IU per day. Overall, the "right" level of vitamin A in the diet is a complex function of many variables (age, size, sex, genetics, and lifestyle, including smoking habits). With a balanced diet, some of which is vitamin A-enriched — for example, skim milk, which contains added vitamin A equal to the amount that is lost during the removal of fat from whole milk — vitamin A deficiency is almost never a problem in the developed world. Exceptions include alcoholics with poor diets, since alcohol interferes with the uptake of vitamin A and with the conversion of retinol to retinoic acid. There are also rare genetic conditions in which vitamin A metabolism is perturbed. In the developed world generally, however, diets provide enough vitamin A.

Given that too much vitamin A can be toxic, how much preformed vitamin A is in plant foods such as spinach, carrots, or orange sweet potatoes? And should we be worried about consuming too many carrots, for example? The answers are "none" and "no," respectively. Plants contain no preformed vitamin A, but they do contain beta-carotene, which is its non-toxic, provitamin precursor. Beta-carotene is not toxic because its conversion to vitamin A in the body is under feedback control; a high circulating level of vitamin A inhibits the conversion of beta-carotene to retinal in the gut. And although an excess of circulating beta-carotene may cause the skin to take on a yellowish cast (because beta-carotene is yellow-orange), no real harm is done. A report from the European Food Safety Authority mentions that doses of 20–180 milligrams per day of beta-carotene, between 100 and 1,800 times the RDA, have been used to treat patients with erythropoietic photoporphyria,[23] with no signs of toxicity and without the development of abnormally high blood vitamin A levels. The amount of beta-carotene in orange sweet potatoes and carrots is significant, and that beta-carotene is converted to retinol upon

---

23 Erythropoietic photoporphyria is caused by defective haemoglobin synthesis and leads to extreme light sensitivity. Vampires are said to suffer from this affliction.

digestion. However, the conversion is far from 100% efficient. For carrots, it may take about 15 IU of beta-carotene to produce one IU of retinol in the blood, and for spinach that number may be just as high or higher, depending on other dietary factors (122). In practical terms, one medium cooked carrot contains about 13,000 IU of beta-carotene, but after digestion it typically will deliver just under 900 IU of retinol to the blood.[24] If high levels of vitamin A are unhealthy, it makes sense to ask whether provitamin A, such as the beta-carotene found in fruits and vegetable, is a safer way to obtain vitamin A. We will look at this question further in the next chapter, but the answer is undoubtedly "yes."

There is public interest in the question of whether consuming large amounts of vitamin A-containing fruits and vegetables may be beneficial for general health reasons. Indeed, a number of studies have supported the idea that eating more fruits and vegetables reduces the risk of cancer (123). It is therefore logical to wonder whether it is the beta-carotene content of fruits and vegetables that provides protection; mutations leading to cancer can be caused by damage to DNA by reactive oxygen species, and carotenoids like beta-carotene are antioxidants. Observational studies have suggested that people who consume less of the carotenoids in their diet have a higher than average rate of several chronic diseases, including cancer, cardiovascular disease, and age-related macular degeneration (the leading cause of blindness in older adults). But such correlational studies are unreliable and subject to bias. In this case, poverty is one of the strongest correlates of poor health, and poor people, whose diets are more likely to be deficient in one or more vitamins or their precursors, will almost always have other factors that predispose them to poor health. Although the scientists carrying out such studies try to neutralize all lifestyle variables, this is never entirely possible, and in the present case, more rigorous studies show that the hypothesis that antioxidants such as beta-carotene reduce cancer and cardiovascular disease is undoubtedly wrong.

This evidence is found in random, prospective, double-blind, "gold standard" clinical trials, just as it was when the importance of vitamin

---

24 The conversion of dietary provitamin A to functional, circulating retinol is a complex process, and its efficiency is affected by other nutrients.

A in reducing childhood deaths was established in the 1980s. In a study on the effects of beta-carotene and retinol on human cancer and cardio-vascular disease, 18,000 people were randomly divided into groups, one of which was given those compounds in addition to their normal diets, while the other received a placebo. Neither those collecting the data nor the test subjects knew who was in which group (124). After four years, no beneficial effects were seen in the treated group; by contrast, the overall risk of lung cancer was *increased* by 28% in those taking the antioxidants (the risk of other cancers was not affected). Cardiovascular disease risk also increased, by 17%. Several such studies have been carried out, but no significant beneficial effect of antioxidants has been found. The increased risk of lung cancer linked to vitamin A may have mostly resulted from participants who were already at an elevated risk for that disease (smokers, asbestos workers) (124). Interestingly, increased consumption of fruits and vegetables was a preventive factor for lung cancer in people who did not receive beta-carotene and retinol in that study (125). The jury is still out on whether higher consumption of fruits and vegetables reduces cancer in general, and lung cancer in particular, but the evidence suggests it does.

Recent animal studies illustrate how complicated the story on an-tioxidants is. In mice with a genetic predisposition to develop lung tu-mours, the antioxidants N-acetylcysteine and vitamin E *increased* the rate of cancer growth and reduced the survival of mice with tumours (126). The significance of the two compounds is that they operate by different mechanisms, but they have in common that one of their end effects is to reduce the tissue levels of reactive oxygen species — in other words, they are both antioxidants. The results make sense in terms of the recently un-covered actions of antioxidants. While they reduce the levels of reactive oxidative species and thereby protect the growth of normal cells, they also suppress mechanisms that regulate the growth of cancer cells. The antiox-idant carotenoids may very well do the same.

A more recent report, on mice with both lung cancer and skin can-cer, shows that antioxidants increase the mobilization of tumour cells to secondary sites in laboratory animals; this mobilization process is called metastasis and is what usually kills a cancer patient (127). Again, this is not a promising finding in terms of the theory that antioxidants such as beta-carotene provide protection against cancer.

So, despite the food-supplement industry's promotion of antioxidants as anti-cancer agents, and many people's adoption of that belief, there is no evidence to support the benefit of antioxidants, and there is accumulating evidence that they may even worsen the outcome for someone with a high likelihood of developing lung tumours (e.g., a smoker).

Retinoic acid has been used in the experimental treatment of advanced xerophthalmia. Applied locally to an affected eye, it was found to stimulate the healing of the cornea in vitamin A-deficient rats (128). It has been used topically to promote faster healing of the eyes in children with corneas damaged by xerophthalmia (129), although this application is not common. Retinoic acid can reduce wrinkling and damage to skin from ultraviolet (UV) radiation and aging (130-132). Many commercial "anti-wrinkling" creams contain retinol, which is converted to retinoic acid in the skin, since topical retinol is less irritating than retinoic acid. Retinoic acid may reduce aging from UV radiation by enhancing the turnover of epidermal cells; this mechanism is presumably also responsible for the use of retinoids in treating acne, psoriasis, and other skin conditions. However, a dangerously enhanced turnover rate could have been the basis for the toxic effects, including extensive skin peeling, experienced by the Danish travellers in the Arctic who in 1913 unfortunately ate polar bear liver (97).

With a few exceptions, such as self-inflicted malnutrition (e.g., anorexia nervosa, alcoholism), vitamin A deficiency is not a significant first-world problem. It used to be, but not any more. There is little evidence that excess consumption of preformed vitamin A is useful for well-fed children or adults, and it may be harmful. On the other hand, there is no doubt that a deficiency in vitamin A has been responsible for blindness and premature death in millions of children in the developing world. Overcoming such deficiencies is the subject of the next chapter. Achieving the goal of adequate vitamin A levels in children of the developing world is currently more difficult than it needs to be, because of various ideological and logistical factors. This is an area of intense disagreement among some health practitioners and critics, and it is a struggle to keep some avenues of potential resolution open.

Summary: The effects of vitamin A on human health

· Vitamin A is an essential micronutrient found in a number of foods, either preformed (in animal sources of food) or as provitamin A (in certain food plants).

· A chronic deficiency causes nightblindness, xerophthalmia, and death; particularly vulnerable are children under the age of six years and pregnant women.

· It is an "anti-infective" agent, reducing the rates of illness and death from many infectious diseases.

· Deficiencies of other micronutrients (minerals, vitamins) and vitamin A can be synergistic — that is, these deficiencies work together to make things even worse.

· A massive overdose (greater than 100 times the RDA) can cause extreme symptoms, including peeling of the skin, gastrointestinal upset, and occasionally death.

· Amounts in excess of the RDA have no beneficial effect for most people.

· Even moderate amounts in chronic excess (two or three times the RDA, daily, for decades) can lead to more fragile bones in the elderly and an increase in fractures and osteoporosis.

· Altered forms of retinoic acid (e.g., isotretinoin and other drugs used to treat skin disorders) can cause birth defects.

· The symptoms of fetal alcohol spectrum disorder may be caused in part by alcohol interfering with vitamin A metabolism.

· Normal diets in the developed world provide sufficient vitamin A without a need for supplements.

· There is little scientific support for the notion that vitamin A causes birth defects.

· While the consumption of too much preformed vitamin A can cause health problems, foods containing beta-carotene are safe in almost any amounts.

CHAPTER 5

Overcoming Vitamin A Deficiency

Supplementation to overcome vitamin A deficiency

It isn't necessary to shop at Whole Foods to get enough vitamin A in your diet. The average citizen in the developed world obtains enough vitamin A to stay healthy from the average diet, available to people of average means. It will contain a sufficient amount of either preformed vitamin A or provitamin A, usually a mixture of the two. Animal-derived foods, particularly liver and dairy products, contain significant amounts of preformed vitamin A, which largely survives cooking. Dark green leafy plants, such as spinach, and many yellow-orange foods, such as orange sweet potatoes, carrots, and pumpkins, contain provitamin A in the form of carotenoids, which are converted to retinol in the human gut. Pick up a milk carton; if it's whole milk, it will say something like "contains 10% of daily vitamin A requirements." That's about 335 IU of preformed vitamin A per cup — just over 10% of the requirement for a grown man and about 30–35% of what nutritionists think a young child requires. Given that (i) the human liver stores excess vitamin A and releases it as blood levels fall and (ii) the uptake of carotenoids in the gut is controlled by feedback from serum retinol, the vitamin A contained in the diets of most people in the developed world is sufficient, and no conscious supplementation with pills or vitamin A-rich foods is necessary.

But for many poor people living in developing regions, whose diets are unbalanced or otherwise insufficient, that isn't the case. After clinical trials showed, in the early 1980s, that large parts of the world were vitamin A deficient, and that children suffering deficiency were more likely to die than those with adequate diets, it became apparent that any solutions would have to be provided by agencies from the developed world. Slowly, that effort began to mobilize. International organizations, including those of the United Nations, along with private donors and government and non-governmental agencies based in several countries, began to generate programs in various regions, among them South and Southeast Asia, sub-Saharan Africa, and parts of Central America.

The problems in various vitamin A-deficient areas are different; what has become clear is that there is no universal solution, short of a broadly based, nutritionally complete diet for all, which is still only a dream. Adding to the challenge is that vitamin A deficiency seldom exists in isolation; it is usually part of a family of deficiencies in other micronutrients, including one or more of zinc, iron, iodine, and other vitamins.

Micronutrient deficiencies can be addressed in two ways: supplementation and food fortification. The World Health Organisation held a conference in 1958, together with the National Institutes of Health of the United States, which marked the beginning of the UN's involvement in combatting vitamin A deficiency. Partly as a result of that conference, programs have been designed to provide large-dose vitamin A supplements in developing countries since the 1980s. The effort is coordinated by the Global Agency for Vitamin A (GAVA) and supported by the United Nations Children's Fund (UNICEF), which partners with the Micronutrient Initiative, headquartered in Canada. The most commonly used measure of vitamin A deficiency is the concentration of retinol or its esters in the blood. A value below 0.70 micromolar is considered to represent deficiency.[25] Based on this value, UNICEF estimates that one out of every three children living in underdeveloped settings are vitamin A deficient. This represents about 190 million children worldwide.

Organizations involved in global health have used large-dose supplementation to provide vitamin A to millions of people, particularly

25 0.70 micromolar, or 0.70 micromoles per litre, corresponds to about 200 micrograms of retinol, or an equivalent amount of its esters, per litre of blood. A million people with this level of retinol have a total of about two pounds (just under one kilogram) of vitamin A in their blood.

preschool children and mothers, who are at risk of vitamin A deficiency in the developing world. The dosage provided in such programs is typically 200,000 IU twice a year, given as capsules, which is what the Johns Hopkins team gave the Indonesian children in the first clinical test of vitamin A supplementation in 1978. The capsules cost about two cents each, but distributing them increases that to about $1–2 per year per child. And monitoring the distribution is important. Simply making capsules available to people in poor countries is not enough; there need to be workers on the ground, ensuring the capsules are utilized. For example, a program in Laos provided iron tablets to pregnant women (iron deficiency being the most important micronutrient problem in the world), but there was no monitoring, and a subsequent interview established that only 14% of the women had taken them (133).

About 500 million vitamin A capsules are distributed worldwide each year. Although 200,000 IU is a massive dose compared to the daily needs of a child (about 1,000), it isn't toxic because the children are vitamin A deficient at the time they receive the supplement, which means that their livers have a large latent storage capacity for excess retinol. The ideal is to provide two supplements a year, but in some cases, only one dose per year is possible due to limited resources.

Large-dose supplementation is being carried out in some 165 countries worldwide. The Government of Bangladesh instituted its first program in 1973, well before the linkage of vitamin A deficiency to childhood deaths had been established. In 1978, Helen Keller International began to work in that country, and in 1982 it joined the government effort. In 1982, the prevalence of nightblindness in Bangladeshi children 12 to 59 months old was 3.6%; this number decreased to 0.06% by 1996 (134). UNICEF estimates that about 69% of children in areas at risk are being reached by supplementation programs. Perhaps because of the focused concern on the least developed countries, they have a better record of coverage than the average for all low-resource settings (135). For example, in the African country of Chad, one of the poorest in the world, UNICEF estimated that greater than 90% of children were being reached in 2014. When UNICEF began its programs in the late 1990s, the number of children receiving two doses of vitamin A a year was low, but it rapidly increased. Between 1999 and 2004 the number of children receiving two doses went from 16% to 58% in at-risk countries. However, that number has not increased much in the past five years. Levels of childhood xerophthalmia, a measure of a more profound vitamin A deficiency, also decreased early in this period but recently have stopped declining. It is important to keep in mind that although effects on vision are symptoms of vitamin A deficiency, death related to vitamin A deficiency can occur without apparent visual impairment.

While the distribution of vitamin A capsules is an effective and straightforward method of overcoming deficiency, and the cost of the capsules is modest, UNICEF and its partner agencies are urging the governments of affected countries to take up the operational cost of the programs themselves. The money available for running all UN programs has limits, and the demands only increase. Using local resources and people to run nutritional supplement programs also gives them "ownership" and can lead to more effective utilization of resources.

In addition to financial limits, unexpected barriers may suddenly diminish the efficacy of vitamin A capsule programs. In 2014, for example, the Ebola crisis in several African countries threatened progress. Furthermore, it has become apparent that supplementation programs can never saturate the need for vitamin A worldwide, and that such programs are sensitive to issues such as donor fatigue, disruptions caused by epidemic disease, and sometimes opposition from internal sources.

One country in which there is official resistance to certain supplementation programs is India (117). There has been little progress in reducing preschool deaths in India since 1980. This is in contrast to Bangladesh and Nepal, where children's death rates were similar to those of India in 1980 but are now significantly lower. There are estimated to be some two million vitamin A-deficient children in India at present. According to outside experts (13), the lack of progress is due to some Indian authorities who have resisted vitamin A capsule programs. Some influential officials in India feel that supplementation programs should be stopped, and the money saved should be used for other purposes (136). These critics argue that although about eight billion vitamin A capsules have been distributed over the years, there has been no demonstrable reduction in childhood mortality or the number of children with low blood retinol levels (137-139). A massive study of the effects of vitamin A supplementation in India found no reduction in preschool children's deaths from all causes (140). But this study has been heavily criticized, and its conclusions run counter to almost all of the experience in other studies (141, 142). Furthermore, the measured level of vitamin A deficiency in children in India is around 62% (143). Even if the incidence of xerophthalmia has not dropped greatly, that by itself is not a reliable guide to the severity of vitamin A deficiency, as morbidity and mortality can occur even when xerophthalmia is not observed (144).

A specific criticism of vitamin A supplementation in India is that most of the lives saved in the earlier trials were due to children not dying from measles — vitamin A supplementation is generally agreed to reduce deaths in measles outbreaks, as first observed by Ellison in 1932 (70). Critics make the point that immunization against measles is widespread and growing in the developing world, so vitamin A supplementation is no longer needed and is counter-productive because it consumes resources (138). However, the case against this claim includes the observation that in the clinical trial of vitamin A supplementation in Nepal in the 1980s, vitamin A reduced mortality from all causes by 30%, and measles was only responsible for about 4% of children's deaths. Most deaths resulted from wasting malnutrition, diarrhoea, dysentery, and other infections (116).

The opposition to the capsule programs by some Indian health officials has been vigorously criticized by many experts (116), and the WHO sides with those who hold that capsule programs are beneficial and should be continued. GAVA, which was formed by several agencies concerned about vitamin A deficiency, has also weighed in on this issue. GAVA points out that many countries still have high under-five mortality rates, many have vitamin A deficiencies, and the two often go together. While the ideal solution is to have vitamin A provided daily by a good diet, supplementation with high-dose capsules semi-annually has a proven record of benefit in areas where a dietary solution is not yet available.

The Indian "capsule rejectors" suggest that a better solution is to have children eat more fruit and vegetables containing beta-carotene, a solution that is presently unavailable, given the level of poverty and poor dietary resources. By contrast, other Indian experts agree with the international consensus that vitamin A deficiency is still a health problem and that, in the absence of better solutions, a high-dose capsule program is required (145). As a result of various factors, it is estimated that only 20% of children in India are covered by vitamin A supplementation programs, even though 62% of them are deficient (143).

Today, it would be difficult to provide new proof that capsule supplementation programs work. Since clinical trials in the past showed that vitamin A supplementation profoundly reduced childhood deaths from all causes in developing world countries, it would be unethical to carry out placebo-control studies; you can't deny some children a treatment that the expert consensus holds to be essential. Because conditions are fluid — with nutritional situations in some countries slowly improving (although often not enough to completely prevent xerophthalmia) and local events (such as Ebola) disrupting whole societies — it is not possible to prove that capsule programs do or don't work as well as they are expected to in individual countries. But the earlier evidence is still considered valid.

Fortifying food to overcome micronutrient deficiency

The other approach to overcoming a micronutrient deficiency is fortification, by one of two ways. The simplest is "industrial fortification," in which a missing micronutrient is added as a pure chemical to a food that will be consumed by the population at risk. This kind of fortification has a history of success with some micronutrients but carries a fundamental requirement: to benefit, people need to purchase or otherwise obtain enough of the fortified food on a regular basis. This usually means that the fortified food must be processed by a central agency and distributed. If the processed food is not affordable, or is not broadly enough consumed, industrial fortification isn't effective. Supplying a micronutrient in foods that are usually grown by many people for themselves, rather than obtained from a central source, will not work for industrial fortification.

One of the earliest successful industrial fortification schemes was a method for providing vitamin D in milk (24). In the early 1920s, Harry Steenbock and his colleagues obtained a patent for doing that by irradiating milk with ultraviolet light, which converts a steroid in milk fat to vitamin D. This essentially ended rickets in North America and Europe. In that case, the fortification was due to an internal chemical reaction induced by an outside agent. Most fortification schemes don't work that way; instead, they involve adding a missing critical micronutrient to a common component of the diet. Iodine is a good example.

There is a horrific painting in the Prado Museum, in Madrid, created by Francisco Goya between 1819 and 1823, called "The Great He-Goat: Witches' Sabbath."[26] In it, a large group of frightening and frightened humans sit in a circle, communing with each other and, apparently, otherworldly spirits. The circle is presided over by the dark figure of a male goat, representing the devil. Many of the people in the painting show signs of a condition called cretinism, which includes mental retardation, distorted facial features, and a grossly enlarged thyroid gland, or goiter. This condition was well known historically, particularly in Spain. Sponge and dried seaweed had been used to treat it for centuries, and in 1813 the Swiss physician Coindet hypothesized that seaweed's therapeutic value was due to it containing the newly discovered element iodine, which he thought was missing in those afflicted with goiter. In 1851, a French chemist again proposed that iodine deficiency was the cause of goiter, and by 1896, iodine was shown to be present in the thyroid, with "cretins" suffering from goiter having less of it than healthy people. The use of iodine supplementation to prevent goiter and cretinism was firmly established when Switzerland, which had a high level of goiter, became the first country to introduce an iodized salt program, in 1922 (146). This essentially eliminated the condition in Switzerland, and the United States followed

---

26 Goya did not title this painting, which he produced as part of a series of gruesome works during his "Black Period." They were painted on the plaster walls of his house, then later transferred to canvas frames and named by other people. There is a different painting titled "Witches' Sabbath" in the Museo Lázaro Galdiano. This museum is also in Madrid.

this lead later that year, thereby eliminating a high rate of goiter in the Midwestern states.

Humans need iodine to maintain the health and function of their thyroid glands. These glands produce the hormones thyroxin and tri-iodothyronine, which help regulate the body's energy metabolism and its early development, among other functions. Synthesis of the thyroid hormones requires iodine, because it is an essential part of their chemical structures. Once synthesized, the thyroid hormones are exported into the bloodstream and distributed. The thyroid hormones regulate the expression of specific genes, much as retinoic acid does, although the target genes are different. Where iodine is absent from the soil, which can be the case in inland areas, people are susceptible to hypothyroidism and goiter. Without enough of the thyroid hormones, the developing human foetus may suffer varying degrees of cognitive disabilities and poor physical development.

The condition of many of the people in Goya's painting was endemic in parts of Spain during his time and, indeed, for an unconscionably long time afterwards. It resulted from iodine insufficiency, due to iodine-poor soil. Remarkably, it was not overcome in that country until the mid-1980s, by the simple expedient of providing iodized salt. In 1922, a prominent Spanish endocrinologist named Marañon pointed out a high level of hypothyroidism and cretinism in people living near the Spanish–Portuguese border. Other scientists showed that rats fed local diets from goiter-prone areas of the country also developed goiter, and that this condition was prevented by providing iodine in the diet. Furthermore, the role of iodine was known from experiences in Switzerland and the United States, which had both just moved to introduce iodized salt. But Marañon decided that the real solution for Spain lay in improving socio-economic conditions, a similar opinion to that held by opponents of vitamin A supplementation in India today (13). The opinion of Marañon, who had strong ties to the monarchy and then, after 1936, the dictator Francisco Franco, was so influential that essentially nothing was done.

Marañon was a brilliant and productive physiologist, but in this matter he was wrong. In 1971, a study found that the prevalence of goiter correlated inversely with the content of iodine in the drinking water in various parts of the country. Despite this, the influence of Marañon (who died in 1960) remained so great that simple fortification of table salt was resisted for decades afterwards. (It didn't help that Franco, who died in 1975, refused to acknowledge the problem's existence.) Finally, a study by the European Thyroid Association in 1985 showed that in the highland region of Las Hurdes, the prevalence of schoolchildren with goiter was 86%; iodized salt was finally made available throughout Spain, and the problem gradually disappeared.

Iodine deficiency, the cause of hypothyroidism, has not been universally eradicated. In 2007, the WHO estimated that two billion people in the world had insufficient iodine intake, and it remains a serious problem in 25 countries. Yet it is a deficiency that is easily prevented. Iodized table salt, in which an iodide ion occasionally replaces a chloride ion (about 20 iodides per million salt molecules), is a cheap and effective answer. It represents probably the most effective example of industrial fortification of a micronutrient.

Although iodized salt cured the goiter problem in Switzerland, America, and eventually Spain (as well as the rest of the developed world wherever iodine deficiency was a problem), like almost all stories to do with nutrition, it still elicits some contrarian views. There are those who claim that there's so little iodine in iodized salt (it evaporates with time) that it serves no useful purpose. Some also claim that in the first world, diets contribute enough iodine that iodized salt is no longer needed. This is probably true, but for the developing world, the argument has no validity. Iodine deficiency exists, and fortification schemes easily eradicate it. The important fact is that almost half of the poorest countries in the world have iodine-deficient soil and lack programs that provide iodized salt or oil in the diet.

Although fortification can work, it can also be risky. Folate — the vitamin first uncovered by Dr. Lucy Wills in her study of fatal anaemia in malnourished, pregnant Indian women — is required for blood formation and for normal growth and development during pregnancy. A precursor, folic acid, has been provided in fortified foods such as white flour in the

United States and Canada since 1996 and 1998, respectively. Adding folic acid to flour was intended to prevent neural tube-related birth defects, the best known of which is spina bifida (before fortification, its prevalence in the United States was seven cases per 10,000 births). New Zealand has recently made folic acid fortification mandatory, and England is considering doing so. One potential problem is that elevated folic acid intake can impair the effectiveness of anti-folate medications used to treat malaria, rheumatoid arthritis, and cancer. It may also inhibit one arm of the immune system, reducing resistance to disease (147). Some evidence exists that excess folate might be present in the blood of a pregnant woman who has an adequate folate level from her diet and then takes vitamin supplements containing folate. There is also evidence that taking folic acid supplements is associated with increased rates of cancer and death from all causes, at least in Norwegian patients with ischemic heart disease. Some researchers considering the risks and benefits in Britain have estimated that for every neural-tube birth defect prevented by adding folic acid to flour, between 370,000 and 780,000 people would be exposed to elevated folate levels (148). A better way to prevent spina bifida and other birth defects due to folate deficiency might be to provide it as a supplement to the mother. But because folate deficiency has its damaging effects early in pregnancy, the folate would need to be in the mother's system before she became pregnant, and many pregnancies are unplanned. That concern could be met by having all women of childbearing age taking a folate-containing supplement. The best approach is not yet clear.

The example of folic acid supplementation illustrates a recurring theme when comparing the micronutritional requirements in well-fed, developed populations and those living in developing-world conditions. This has already been noted with respect to vitamin A; children who are relatively healthy may actually be slightly worse off in terms of lower respiratory tract infections if they receive supplemental vitamin A, while those who are initially deficient greatly benefit (113). There can be too much of a good thing, although in the case of vitamin A, there is a safe solution: to provide the provitamin A beta-carotene rather than preformed vitamin A itself. The provitamin is safe at almost any level.

Chemical fortification with vitamin A has been used. In Guatemala, for example, a powdered form of the vitamin A ester retinyl palmitate was added to sugar beginning in 1975 (149). This program decreased the number of children suffering from vitamin A deficiency, as evidenced by their serum retinol levels (150). Almost all children who were below the deficiency threshold of 0.70 micromolar rose above it. The program was stopped in 1979 due to cost, as the vitamin A supplement was being produced by a major pharmaceutical company. The program was restarted in 1987 and has been continued since. Sugar fortification has also been carried out in Honduras and Costa Rica. Sugar is now a major source of vitamin A for infants and young children in those countries, providing about 30% of their daily requirements. Despite the expense of the added vitamin A ester, the overall cost of this type of fortification is low (151).

Other foods have also been fortified with vitamin A, but most such products have not been widely adopted. The key to successful chemical fortification is to choose a substance that is centrally processed and widely enough consumed by the target population, with the most important targets being pregnant women and young children; prominent examples are sugar, salt, and monosodium glutamate. It's important to moderate the total amount of retinol consumed, in whatever form; too much preformed vitamin A (i.e., retinol or its esters) is toxic, and even modest overdoses can lead to a decrease in bone health. This is not the case with biofortification, which provides plants rich in carotenoids, provitamin A. It is almost impossible to over-consume provitamin A in any form available from plants, making biofortification the best choice for adding vitamin A to the diet.

The orange sweet potato as an ideal source of vitamin A

Supplementation and industrial fortification of micronutrients are both designed to provide a missing component of a healthy diet. In fortification with a pure chemical, the component is added to a food, whereas in supplementation, a micronutrient is provided in pure form, often as a pill or liquid. But these methods are incomplete, as seen by the fact that fewer than 70% of the world's children receive vitamin A supplementation. Another approach complements or replaces supplementation: biofortification with a food containing the desired micronutrient. Fortunately, one food — the orange sweet potato — is almost ideal for this purpose as far as vitamin A is concerned, and it is being used to address vitamin A deficiencies in sub-Saharan Africa.

New Vision advertises itself as Uganda's leading daily newspaper. Published in the capital city, Kampala, it has a circulation of between 35,000 and 40,000. On October 2, 2013, it featured a story about a boy named Yovani Bagirewa, aged one and a half years, who had been suffering from frequent bouts of ill health. His parents thought he might be a victim of witchcraft exercised by neighbours with whom they were having an argument about a property deal. His parents visited shrines and hospitals, to little effect. Yovani lost his appetite, suffered attacks of diarrhoea, and lost weight. His mother sadly related that a touch to his legs would make him scream. Then, he came down with measles. Enlightened medical staff advised his parents to give him foods rich in vitamin A. Fortunately, Yovani and his parents lived in a village, Bukokoba, where they could get the orange sweet potato, rich in vitamin A, which promises to help vitamin A-deficient children and their mothers in a wide swathe of sub-Saharan Africa. The orange sweet potato is not native to Uganda or other parts of Africa afflicted by vitamin A deficiency. Farmers there grow the white sweet potato, which doesn't have significant amounts of vitamin A. But the orange version has been brought to the continent and planted in farms around numerous villages in Uganda, Mozambique, and other countries. This has made inroads against vitamin A deficiency, which afflicts millions of African children and kills hundreds of thousands each year, according to the best estimates. Once he began to consume orange sweet potato, Yovani soon regained his health. That may have been coincidental, but it fits the pattern of what has been happening in sub-Saharan Africa in the past decade.

There are sweet potatoes and there are yams, and they are about as distantly related as two flowering plants can be. Also, despite their names, the sweet potato and the round, Irish, or solanum potato have little in common; the sweet potato belongs to the same family as the morning glory and a number of poisonous cousins. Many people think that orange sweet potatoes are yams because they are somewhat similar in shape and size, and some grocery stores, particularly in North America, call them that (yam fries are really "orange sweet potato fries"). Sweet potatoes come in a variety of colours, and most grocery stores stock both a pale yellow variety and a deep orange one. Yams also come in a variety of colours, but they are starchier and drier, and are mostly grown in sub-Saharan Africa, where they are a dietary mainstay in many countries. They are not common in North American grocery stores. There is also a profound difference in the content of vitamin A between orange sweet potatoes and yams: the orange (but not the pale white) sweet potato is one of the richest food sources of provitamin A (beta-carotene), while the yam contains almost none. The colour of orange sweet potatoes — which exist in dozens of varieties — reflects their content of beta-carotene, just as it does for carrots. The darker the orange, the higher the beta-carotene content.

Carrots and orange sweet potatoes, two of the most beta-carotene-rich vegetables known, began their roles in human nutrition worlds apart. The carrot was first seen in Europe in the Middle Ages and was subsequently developed there to become the edible root of today. Its ancestor is thought to be the wild carrot, a bitter, purple or yellow, spindly, multi-rooted plant; we have evidence of its existence thousands of years ago in Asia and the Middle East. The evolutionary path from wild to domesticated carrots has not been thoroughly traced. But by selecting from existing yellow carrots for a deeper orange colour, Dutch and French growers, beginning some time before the 16th century, produced carrots that have a high level of beta-carotene. The art of that period and later times often shows examples of the various stages of colour development in one picture, from pale yellow to orange. At the same time, growers selected for the more robust, thicker, single root.[27]

The origin of the other champion of beta-carotene content, the orange sweet potato, has been traced to Latin America. Upon digestion, the beta-carotene of orange sweet potatoes is converted to retinal and

---

27 There is a myth that Dutch breeders developed carrots with a deep orange colour to honour the royal House of Orange of that country in the 16th century. Experts on the history of the carrot think there is no evidence for this.

then to retinol or its esters. Theoretically, one microgram of beta-carotene could give rise to one microgram of retinol, but in practice, it's less. A modest fraction of the beta-carotene in foods is lost on cooking. But the uptake of beta-carotene in the gut, and its conversion to preformed vitamin A, is always significantly less than the theoretical limit. In part, this is because the higher the level of circulating retinol, the lower the efficiency of beta-carotene digestion. This feedback keeps us safe from an overdose of vitamin A derived from beta-carotene. But the efficiency of digesting vitamin A is also affected by the rest of the diet. For example, a diet deficient in fat leads to poorer digestion of beta-carotene and other carotenoids, even if the need for vitamin A is high. Fortunately, even a moderate amount of fat (for example, cooking oil) increases the efficiency. Preformed vitamin A supplements (retinol) in oil, as provided by vitamin A supplementation programs, are highly efficient at increasing circulating amounts of retinol or retinyl esters.

A typical medium-sized orange sweet potato contains around 22,000 IU of beta-carotene, but after being cooked and eaten it may deliver only about 1,700 IU of retinol to the blood. In other words, it takes 13 units of beta-carotene in the original raw sweet potato to provide 1 unit of retinol in the body. This was the level of conversion observed in Bangladeshi men, many of whom were relatively deficient in vitamin A and lived on sub-optimal diets (152). But the conversion efficiency varies widely, depending on what else is being consumed as well as the individual's health and dietary circumstances (153). The ratio established by the Institute of Medicine in the United States is 12:1 in a mixed diet, but this improves to 2:1 in oil, which corresponds to oil-based capsules of pure beta-carotene. The same report estimated an efficiency of conversion ranging from 9:1 to 28:1 for beta-carotene in a typical developing world diet. Other studies have found the bioconversion of beta-carotene in maize (corn) to be as high as 3.2:1 if it is present in a diet with adequate oil content (154). It's a complex dietary issue.

The RDAs for vitamin A in the United States are 3,000 IU for an adult male, 2,300 IU for an adult female, and 1,000 IU for a child aged three to four years. In the example of the orange sweet potato above, where one medium potato delivered 1,700 IU of retinol, it provided about half of what an adult male requires daily but was easily enough to sustain a child. And if the child were to consume more beta-carotene than the RDA, no harm would arise, as its conversion to retinol in the gut is regulated, in a feedback loop, by the existing blood levels.

The efficiency of converting beta-carotene in the plant to retinol in the body is similar for spinach. However, spinach is a relatively low-density source of beta-carotene — a cup of raw spinach, about the amount that might be found in a large salad, contains under 3,000 IU of beta-carotene. Not insignificant, certainly, but not an answer to the problems of African children like Yovani; growing enough spinach to overcome their vitamin A deficiency would require vast quantities of arable land and water and would not provide the other huge benefit of the sweet potato, which is that it contains a lot of food energy. There may be another problem in obtaining beta-carotene from spinach: studies have shown only a trivial increase in the blood levels of retinol and beta-carotene when spinach was added to the diet of villagers in Java, whereas the identical amount of beta-carotene in wafers increased those levels significantly (155). Part of the problem probably resulted from other dietary circumstances — for example, spinach's low fat content.

The orange sweet potato appears to be an almost ideal answer to the problems of vitamin A-deficient diets in poor African countries. In many such nations, people have been growing and eating sweet potatoes for hundreds of years, although they are not indigenous. (They may have been introduced from America by returning slave traders.) The sweet potatoes being grown before the end of the 20th century were almost exclusively white-fleshed, which contain almost no beta-carotene. The orange sweet potato, brought from America in the past few decades, did increase the vitamin A status of poor children in South Africa (156). It is also one of the most productive crops per acre, even on poor soils, provided there is at least some rain. It can tolerate dry spells and is relatively, although not entirely, disease resistant. But to succeed, orange sweet potato programs need to address a number of issues, and these have required intense research and development work.

In the first place, the productivity of the orange sweet potato must be at least as good as, and preferably better than, the existing white-fleshed ones, otherwise farmers may be reluctant to make the switch. In the past few years, breeding programs in Africa have produced dozens of varieties of orange sweet potatoes, beginning with a collection of seeds from around the world, to identify high-yielding varieties. There are infectious agents, principally viruses, that target sweet potatoes, reducing yield. Some areas of Africa have two rainy seasons and two resulting harvest cycles; they therefore can grow sweet potatoes for enough of the year to provide adequate vitamin A. But some have a single rainy season, and storage of orange sweet potatoes can be a problem (although techniques for doing that have been developed). The distribution of the potato stock is more complicated than it is for some crops. The programs distribute vine cuttings, which are used by farmers to start and maintain their own crops. The process of distribution is somewhat cumbersome, as the sacks of vines are heavy. Finally, a kind of reverse socio-economic status issue can interfere with progress. As farmers become more prosperous, and as people move into cities, they tend to eat less and less sweet potato, preferring grains and other foods. This is not unusual; the same phenomenon took place earlier in the 20th century in the United States, where today's per capita consumption of sweet potatoes is about 10% of what it was in 1900, even though it is by any measure one of the healthiest of vegetables to eat. China has recently undergone a similar decline in sweet potato consumption, decreasing by 56% between 1963 and 2003. This is a significant issue, because vitamin A deficiency is still an important nutritional problem in China.

Programs to introduce orange sweet potatoes are poised to help eliminate, or at least greatly reduce, the problem of vitamin A deficiency in sub-Saharan Africa. But to provide benefit, three conditions need to be met (157): (i) the required plant must be adapted to the areas concerned, which in this case have different growing conditions across the affected parts of Africa; (ii) the nutritional efficacy of the crop plant must be established; and (iii) people must be willing to make changes to their farming and dietary customs to incorporate it into their lives. Each of these conditions is being addressed for orange sweet potatoes in Africa.

Early results have indicated the need for more drought-resistant varieties, which could be obtained by crossing the introduced orange sweet potatoes (obtained from many parts of the world, with one of the best performing being "Resisto" from the United States) with local varieties of white sweet potatoes, already known to perform well under local conditions. Then, the nutritional value of the chosen varieties must be established. Do they improve vitamin A status under local conditions, and will people grow and eat them? For example, a less sweet variety is being developed to appeal to the taste of people in Ghana. Finally, to achieve sufficient production, conditions that will reward growing and selling in the local market must be considered.

The history of the orange sweet potato in Africa involves a veritable alphabet soup of agencies, some indigenous to Africa, some originating elsewhere, all striving to reduce deficiencies in vitamin A and other micronutrients on that continent. The agency most directly involved in baby Yovani Bagirewa's case is the Volunteer Efforts for Development Concerns (VEDCO), an indigenous NGO. In addition to the orange sweet potato, VEDCO also distributes an iron-rich bean, iron being another of the essential micronutrients that children of the developing world often lack (the three most required micronutrients are iron, vitamin A, and zinc).

The growing interest in projects directed at using the orange sweet potato in Africa follows demonstrations that such an approach can work. In 2003–2004, a study in a resource-poor part of Mozambique showed that the intake and retinol levels of children were increased by the growth and consumption of orange sweet potatoes (158). This occurred despite very poor sanitary and health conditions, malnutrition, and morbidity. In places where people are poor, such as the study area in Mozambique, it is difficult to determine the effectiveness of the sweet potato because of high levels of childhood illness. Children suffering from recurrent diarrhoea, for example, do not retain either the macronutrients (calories) or micronutrient (beta-carotene) of the sweet potato. However, increasing vitamin A levels by introducing the orange sweet potato did reduce morbidity from diarrhoea in Mozambique (159). Further, people were happy to grow and eat the orange-fleshed potato instead of the white varieties they had been growing before (in fact, children in Mozambique somewhat preferred the sweeter orange variety).

Uganda also has a high rate of vitamin A deficiency, and although a capsule supplementation program has been pursued there, the coverage achieved has been estimated to be under 67%. (Reports on the ground suggest that often the official numbers are over-estimates. Remote and poor areas, in particular, are less likely to receive and benefit from such programs.) In 2007, the organization HarvestPlus initiated a project to provide orange sweet potato vines to farmers in Uganda.[28] Between 2007 and 2009, HarvestPlus and its partners distributed orange sweet potatoes to more than 24,000 households in Mozambique and Uganda. In 2012, the results of this intervention showed that in both countries, as in the previous test in Mozambique, the cultivated orange sweet potatoes improved the vitamin A status of women and children (160). HarvestPlus estimates that consumption of biofortified orange sweet potatoes in Uganda could eliminate 40–66% of the burden of vitamin A deficiency, as measured by disability-adjusted life years (a standard measure of impact, calculated to determine the number of years lost to poor health, disability, or death) (157). People were informed that consumption of the orange sweet potato would protect their children from vitamin A deficiency, and that it grew just as well as the previously cultivated white version. If anything, the colour seemed to be an attractive feature to consumers, who are willing to pay a premium for the orange potato. Acceptance of the orange sweet potato in Uganda and Mozambique was 61% and 68%, respectively, within two years of introduction (158, 160).

The orange sweet potato programs in Africa depend heavily on the participation of women. Women do most of the sweet potato farming, and they dominate the numbers of farmers receiving potato planting stock; HarvestPlus estimates that more than 70% of the farmers they provide with planting material are women. From the beginning, dissemination of information on the nutrition and farming of orange sweet potatoes has been an intrinsic part of programs aimed at introducing it

---

28 HarvestPlus is a creation of two existing international agencies concerned with nutrition in the developing world, with headquarters in Colombia and in Washington, DC.

to countries in Africa, and this educational activity is also run almost entirely by women.

It is unlikely that any single program will eradicate vitamin A deficiency in Africa. The emerging theme is that supplementation and biofortification are both important, and the same lesson undoubtedly applies to other parts of the developing world. Local and regional biofortification targets need to be identified and brought to bear. The next chapter identifies a biofortification approach to vitamin A deficiency that has a much more fraught history, despite its apparent promise.

Biofortification is being actively pursued in many countries of the world, with the focus on numerous food crops in addition to the orange sweet potato being developed in Africa (161). Provitamin A carotenoids are also being developed in bananas and plantains (Uganda, Nigeria, the Congo, and other African countries), cassava (Congo, Nigeria, Brazil), pumpkin (Brazil), rice (Philippines, Indonesia, India), and sorghum (Kenya, Burkina Faso, Nigeria). Plants enriched in iron and zinc include beans (Rwanda, Congo, Brazil), cowpea (India, Brazil), pearl millet (India), rice (Bangladesh, India, Brazil), sorghum (India), and wheat (India, Pakistan, China, Brazil). But progress is slow; development of a new biofortified food crop can take six to 10 years once a path has been identified. Two different strategic models of biofortification are used, depending on the nutritional patterns of a country. In the African countries involved in programs for vitamin A and other micronutrients, biofortification is largely focused on a small number of staple nutrients consumed by almost all people in a given area, an example being the sweet potato. Brazil, where there are several staple crops, employs a different strategy — biofortification is being developed in a "food basket" of crops, reflecting that nation's broader consumption pattern.

Supplementation, using vitamin A capsules, and industrial fortification, as carried out in Guatemala and other Latin American countries with the addition of vitamin A palmitate to sugar, are both "top-down" approaches. They involve factories located in the developed world or in cities of that developing country. The material then flows into the less developed world or into the countryside, respectively. Biofortification, as seen in the orange sweet potato programs in Africa, is different. Although this solution initially depends on intervention via programs operated by NGOs and universities, often from the developed world, once in place the solution flows from the countryside to the rest of the population, including the cities. When mature, it is a bottom-up scheme — one that ideally comes close to sustaining itself once it's working, with some expenditures being required for monitoring and maintenance. Funding organizations such as the Clinton Global Initiative and the Bill and Melinda Gates Foundation are important for the development and early guidance of biofortification programs in the developing world, and they have contributed heavily. But once programs are fully operational they should be self-sustaining; in fact, they should return wealth to the larger community.

The complexity of the work going on in different parts of the developing world is evident. Policy must follow the science and must consider the societies of the affected people. Unanticipated issues and developments arise and must be approached in a rational way. Programs to optimize biofortification and supplementation of micronutrients such as vitamin A need to contain components that evaluate benefits and risks, and they must identify factors in the affected populations that can influence the outcomes. This is recognized by organizations such as HarvestPlus, for which education is an essential component of programs to provide the orange sweet potato in sub-Saharan Africa.

Given the care and attention to science that is accompanying the best programs for providing micronutrients in the developing world, it is discouraging to see the data-free, often irrational nature of nutritional information churned out on web sites and television programs in the developed world. One of the greatest frustrations for nutritional scientists is to witness the hysterical and unsubstantiated opposition to a potentially important development of another biofortification scheme for the developing world. That story — which is also about vitamin A but carries lessons for other nutritional developments as well — is the subject of the next chapter.

CHAPTER 6

Golden Rice:
Brilliance and Confusion

The rice-dependent world needs a solution

Capsules containing high doses of preformed vitamin A, and orange sweet potatoes, provide remedies for vitamin A deficiency for much of the developing world. They are straightforward solutions that complement each other in parts of sub-Saharan Africa, and may someday help eradicate vitamin A deficiency there. But they are not a universal solution. Large swaths of Southeast and South Asia are plagued by vitamin A deficiency, but the orange sweet potato is not a useful complement to capsule programs in those regions. Most of these countries are part of the rice-dependent world, in which three billion people depend on rice for as much as 80% of their daily calories. Rice provides the greatest agricultural yield and monetary return per acre of any grain, and poor farmers in rice-growing regions do not have the option of abandoning it for the orange sweet potato.[29] There is also the problem of storage; while farmers in parts of Africa have methods for storing sweet potatoes, new strategies would have to be worked out for other parts of the tropical and sub-tropical world. There is presently no natural crop that can provide an effective backup for capsule supplementation programs in most of the countries affected by vitamin A deficiency.

---

29 Rice yields of four tons per acre and higher are not unusual. Although more acreage in the world is planted with wheat, its yield is usually below two tons per acre.

The ideal solution would be to find a type of rice containing adequate levels of beta-carotene in its seed. Unfortunately, in decades of searching, nobody has yet uncovered such a rice strain; unlike the orange sweet potato, rice provides no natural solution to vitamin A deficiency. There is, however, a potential solution, and like the sweet potato-based programs in Africa, it depends on the development of a staple, vitamin A-rich food. It has the advantages that it can become sustainable and almost free for its users. But it also has a major disadvantage, because it takes the form of a genetically engineered rice that contains a high level of beta-carotene. This is the famous, or infamous, "Golden Rice," and in addition to reflecting advances in science and technology, its history also features another modern trend: the opposition to such advances when they involve the genetic engineering (GE) of food plants. To put it mildly, Golden Rice has generated a strong negative response in some parts of the world. A generic opposition to GE, largely originating in the wealthy and well-fed developed world, hinders the advancement of this technology to solve a range of some of the most important nutritional problems in the developing world, including the provision of micronutrients, and resistance to drought and plant diseases.

Genetic modification can arise through a number of techniques, including hybridization (crossing two different strains of the same organism) and forced mutation using mutagenic chemicals or irradiation with X-rays or UV light. Genetic engineering refers to a directed change of the genetic blueprint of an organism using the techniques of molecular biology, and is also a form of genetic modification.

Beta-carotene gives the fruit of a plant a yellow or orange colour. There are a few coloured strains of rice in the world, including a Red Rice that has been cultivated in Bhutan for thousands of years and a Brown Jasmine Rice in Cambodia, but there is no rice that produces vitamin A in its endosperm — the part of the rice seed that remains after rice is milled. The pigments in the Red and Brown Jasmine rices are not directly related to beta-carotene and are not precursors of vitamin A. Rice bran (the outer layer of the rice seed) contains minute quantities of beta-carotene (162), but it would require eating 20–40 kilograms of rice bran (44–88 pounds) to provide the RDA for beta-carotene, and about seven times that weight of brown rice itself. Rice does produce significant quantities of beta-carotene in its leaves, but humans can't digest these. Nonetheless, this indicates that the genes necessary to produce it are present in the rice genome, although they are not expressed in the endosperm.

The invention of genetic engineering of plants

Golden Rice was developed to create rice with a useful level of beta-carotene in its endosperm. The history of its design and creation began with tobacco plants and can be traced back to 1983, an important year for plant molecular biology. At a scientific meeting in Miami in January of that year, three research groups reported the creation of genetically engineered plants, the details of which they subsequently published in peer-reviewed journals (163-165). What all three groups created was GE tobacco, the plant molecular biologist's favourite subject. (Tobacco cells are relatively easy to transform with foreign DNA and then grow into complete plants.) One group was in Belgium, and two were in St. Louis, Missouri. This flurry of activity followed a chapter in plant biology that had begun in 1976, when some of the same scientists discovered the mechanism by which tobacco plants develop a disease called crown gall. In this condition, bacteria infect a tobacco plant through a wound, and soon a large growth, teeming with bacteria, appears on the plant. What scientists in Seattle, Washington, led by Dr. Mary Dell Chilton, and in Ghent, Belgium, headed by Drs. Mark van Montagu and Jozef Schell, discovered was that the bacteria, *Agrobacterium tumafaciens*, were injecting a large, circular piece of DNA, called a plasmid, into the plant cell's nucleus. There it took the tobacco plant's genome hostage and forced it to produce a plant growth hormone. The result was a surge of growth, culminating in a large tumour, a crown gall, filled with bacteria.

What intrigued both groups about the mechanism of crown gall was that this method of taking over a cell's genetic output was very similar to what had been discovered a few years earlier by two California scientists, Stanley Cohen and Herbert Boyer. Cohen and Boyer knew that the common gut bacterium *E. coli* has plasmids that individual cells can share with each other. Sometimes a bacterial cell containing a DNA plasmid establishes close contact with another one and passes a copy of the plasmid into it, thereby genetically transforming the recipient cell (this is referred to as "bacterial sex"). This discovery was medically significant because plasmids often carry genes for antibiotic resistance, and they are an important mechanism for its spread. Cohen and Boyer wanted to see whether they could use plasmid DNA to transfer other genes into bacterial cells. They inserted foreign DNA into a bacterial plasmid's DNA, forced bacteria to take up this "recombinant DNA," and tested for genetic transfer. They found that, indeed, cells that had taken up the recombinant DNA plasmid were genetically transformed; they were the first products of genetic engineering.

Cloning using recombinant DNA in bacteria was immediately useful in basic research, and also had practical applications. For example, recombinant DNA in bacterial (or yeast) cells is the source of essentially all of the insulin used today. Before GE, diabetics had to take bovine or porcine insulin, purified from pancreases obtained from slaughterhouses. In addition to involving a messy and costly process, the animal-derived insulin could sometimes elicit a reaction from the diabetic's immune system, which almost never happens with recombinant human insulin (and if it does, there are ways to overcome the problem). The fact that insulin-producing bacteria or yeast contain genes of both human and bacterial (or yeast) origin initially caused concern, for both scientists and the public, but after risk assessment and extensive testing, they were found not to be biohazardous — i.e., not harmful to humans or the environment.

With their discovery that crown gall disease in tobacco is caused by a plant bacterial plasmid, Chilton, von Montagu, Schell, and their colleagues had uncovered in the plant world something similar to plasmids that are shared between bacteria. The obvious question was, could plants be genetically engineered using the plasmids of *Agrobacteria* as the transforming mechanism? The answer, which took seven years of intense labour by dozens of scientist in both laboratories, was "yes." A foreign piece of DNA, a gene, could be transferred into many kinds of plant cells if it was inserted into the genome of the *Agrobacterium tumafaciens* plasmid that caused the crown gall disease Pasteur famously declared that chance favours the prepared mind; these investigators were successful because they were lucky enough to be working with the only bacterial species, *Agrobacterium*, that is able to genetically transform plant cells with their plasmids. (Transformation with *Agrobacterial* DNA is not an unnatural event. In 2015 it was discovered that all cultivars of the domesticated sweet potato have been transformed by *Agrobacterial* DNA [166].)

Chilton had moved to Washington University, in St. Louis, in 1979. By 1983, her group, another one in St. Louis, and a third in Belgium had succeeded in transferring into a tobacco plant a gene that wasn't part of either the bacterial or the plasmid genomes. The transferred gene became part of the plant's genome and directed the production of a new protein. All three reported their success at the fateful meeting in January of that year and soon published their results in detail (163-165). Plant genetic engineering had begun.

It was no accident that two research groups focused on plant GE were in St. Louis. One of the groups was working in the research laboratory of Monsanto, the chemical company headquartered there. But Monsanto was so eager to get in on the anticipated action in plant biotechnology that it was also providing part of the support for Chilton's research. And, not wanting to miss any chances, it also funded the rival group in Belgium. Later in 1983, Chilton took a position at the CIBA-Geigy Corporation in Switzerland, which, after a couple of rounds of mergers, became Syngenta AG, Monsanto's great European rival, and subsequently a key player in the development of Golden Rice.

By 1984, the potential of plant GE had caught the attention of research directors at the Rockefeller Foundation, which, together with the Ford Foundation, had been the original sponsors of the International Rice Research Institute (IRRI), established in Manila in 1960. The IRRI was tasked with creating better varieties of rice to address food shortages in the developing world. In just a few years, IRRI scientists had cultivated one of the first products of the "Green Revolution" in rice production. This was a hybrid rice called IR8, which had greatly improved growth properties (it stayed upright when older varieties might fall over in a high wind or heavy rain), and vastly improved yields, even with low levels of fertilizer. The initial steps of creating IR8 were overseen by an American scientist named Peter Jennings, who had selected the eighth seedling (hence IR8) of the 38th cross-fertilization as the plant on which to carry out further selection. All of this work was done using conventional genetics, which has been improving agricultural crops since the beginning of their cultivation by humans some 10,000 years ago.

Jennings had been working for the Rockefeller Institute in Mexico and Colombia for four years when he went to the IRRI to become a rice breeder. All the time that he was involved in the development of the new strains of high-yield rice, he was nagged by the desire to find a type of rice that produced beta-carotene in its endosperm. He was aware of the vision problems caused by vitamin A deficiency, which were endemic in many resource-poor countries heavily dependent on rice as their staple food. A rice that provided beta-carotene, provitamin A, might solve the deficiency. But in his travels and work in various parts of the world, he had not found such a plant. Although unpolished, brown rice is nutritionally better because it provides some of the water-soluble B vitamins, it also contains only microscopic amounts of beta-carotene, and eating unpolished rice is not a solution to the problem of vitamin A deficiency. In 20 years, Jennings had not found a rice that contained beta-carotene in its endosperm; it probably doesn't exist in nature. The Rockefeller Foundation supported the search, as well as attempts to find or develop it in global collections of rice seed, or by mutating millions of rice seeds. All to no avail.

The invention of Golden Rice

The directors of research programs at the Rockefeller Foundation were aware of the invention of plant GE in 1983, and they thought that this development might provide a way to address some of the world's pressing nutritional needs. To that end, they organized a meeting, the first one of the foundation's International Program on Rice Biotechnology, which was held at the IRRI, in Manila, in 1984. One evening over beers, after the day's formal sessions were finished, Gary Toenniessen, who was the foundation's director in charge of its rice biotechnology program, informally asked the scientists: "Which gene would you pick to put into rice by GE, if that could be done? What is your favourite trait?" The plant breeders attending mainly came from conventional backgrounds. Although they were certainly aware of the development of GE plants, most were not personally familiar with the technology, and many were frankly sceptical about it. It was a little like asking a room full of symphony orchestra conductors, relaxing post-prandially, which hip-hop tune they might see themselves conducting at their next performance. But the rice scientists were game, and ideas related to disease immunity or drought resistance were brought up. Then it was the turn of Peter Jennings, creator of IR8. The room leaned forward to hear his idea. His laconic comment: "Yellow endosperm." Some of his fellow scientists exchanged puzzled glances. Jennings explained that the colour yellow in a plant usually means that it contains beta-carotene, and that for years he had been searching, fruitlessly, for a natural rice with this feature. He was aware of the health problems caused by vitamin A deficiency in many poor countries and also that rice is often the main food in those places.

The directors of the Rockefeller Foundation thought the idea of using GE to produce rice that contained beta-carotene might have merit, and it began supporting work toward this goal. The foundation underwrote research projects aimed at understanding how beta-carotene is synthesized in the leaves of the rice plant, in hopes that this might illuminate a pathway for producing it in the endosperm. The urgency of the project increased when the evidence from clinical trials, first those of Sommer's group and then confirmatory ones, demonstrated that vitamin A was important not only for vision but also to reduce the number of children dying of all causes. This was consistent with what had been seen in the 1920s and 1930s by British doctors who had dubbed vitamin A the "anti-infective agent" (68, 70). Alfred Sommer's epiphany during the Christmas week of 1982, described in Chapter 1, reignited an appreciation of the more general importance of vitamin A in human health.

After 1985, Toenniessen was responsible for the foundation's International Program on Rice Biotechnology, which to date has invested over 100 million dollars in rice research and development. Although no natural rice with yellow endosperm was discovered, progress was made in understanding the pathway for the biosynthesis of beta-carotene, and in identifying the genes that encode the proteins for this synthesis. Somewhat surprisingly, rice endosperm has most of the enzymes required for beta-carotene synthesis, and also most of the intermediates involved. However, a couple of enzymes are missing. It's like a hiking trail with a washed-out rope bridge.

In 1992, the Rockefeller Foundation sponsored a meeting in New York of parties interested in beta-carotene-containing rice. Dr. Ingo Potrykus, from the Swiss Federal Institute of Technology, in Zürich, and Dr. Peter Beyer, of the University of Freiburg, in Germany, met at that meeting and began discussing how they might collaborate. Soon after, they proposed to the Rockefeller Foundation a research project using GE to generate rice containing beta-carotene in its endosperm. The foundation's scientific advisors thought this would be very difficult, with a good chance of failure, but they supported it anyway.

The problem Potrykus and Beyer faced was that there wasn't just one step missing in the conversion of precursor to beta-carotene — there were five. Several of these steps could probably be carried out by a single enzyme, but still, it was a profoundly challenging problem. Previous plant GE had involved the transfer of just single genes. Beyer was familiar with the pathway of beta-carotene synthesis in daffodils, which gives rise to their lovely yellow colour, so one daffodil gene involved in the pathway was incorporated into a plant plasmid vector. A controlling DNA sequence that would drive its expression in endosperm was coupled to it, as was a "locator" section that would direct the protein produced to enter an intracellular compartment where the rest of the pathway was present. (Plant cells aren't just bags of enzymes. They have compartments.) Another gene needed to rebuild the bridge was similarly engineered. It was a degree of sophistication in plant GE not seen before. Many transformations were attempted before one showed an interesting, novel signal on analysis;

chromatography carried out in Beyer's laboratory in Freiburg showed that there was a new peak,[30] which appeared to correspond to beta-carotene, in one of the transformed rice plants. Beyer quickly went back to look at the rice sample and realized that it had a faint yellowish hue. It was the first beta-carotene-containing rice seed in the world.

Potrykus and Beyer filed a patent for their technology in March of 1999. They sent a manuscript describing their work to the journal *Nature*, in England: the editor declined even to have it reviewed. A few months later they were at a conference in the United States, and a colleague suggested that they immediately send their manuscript to the journal *Science*, in the United States, whose editors published it on January 14, 2000 (167). This provided the "proof of concept," although not yet the needed final product.

The first beta-carotene rice produced only a low level of beta-carotene, but it generated a strong reaction in the world. TIME magazine featured Ingo Potrykus on its cover that summer, with the caption "This Rice Could Save a Million Kids a Year." But just as quickly, a strong negative opinion surfaced, as opponents of GE decried its development. Both admirers and critics were soon referring to it as "Golden Rice," the first group using the term as an accolade, the second using it ironically, as reflecting a chance for the agricultural biotechnology industry to make a lot of money.

Production of the first Golden Rice has been referred to as a "tour de force," in reference to the complexity of technical problems that had to be overcome. It took some 60 scientists, working in two research centres, almost 10 years. But it was far from a finished project. For one thing, the level of beta-carotene was too low to be useful. Greenpeace, which seized on this feature as part of its continuing campaign to discredit the Golden Rice project, claimed that a woman would have to eat 18 kilograms (40

---

30 Chromatography is a workhorse technology for the separation of molecules according to their chemical and physical properties. A mixture of molecules is passed over a medium, often contained in a long, thin tube, and the molecules emerge sequentially. The media used vary widely and perform the separation based on properties such as the size, electrical charge, or water solubility of the molecules in the original mixture. Chromatography existed early in the 20th century, but its application to biochemical research blossomed only in the 1940s. Before chromatography, separation techniques were primitive, as already alluded to in the discussion of the work of vitamin discovery.

pounds) of the prototype Golden Rice to pass on enough to her breastfed baby to do it any good. The term "fool's gold" appeared in critical articles. Although the Greenpeace claim was a great overestimate, the rice would indeed need a higher beta-carotene content to be useful, and that became the goal of subsequent research efforts. Furthermore, the Golden Rice trait would need to be crossed into strains of rice grown in various regions of the developing world to create a suitable source of vitamin A for people living there, and those hybrids would have to be as productive as existing strains.

When Potrykus and Beyer began the Golden Rice project, their goal was to produce a biofortified source of vitamin A that could be freely distributed in the developing world, but now they came up against the barriers standing in the way of creating and giving such a gift. In the first place, they realized that to develop Golden Rice as a practical source of vitamin A (that is, with a higher beta-carotene content) in a reasonable time required technical resources that were beyond their own capabilities. Moreover, some of the technology they had already used, and some they were likely to need, was the intellectual property of large agribusinesses such as Zeneca and Novartis in Europe, Monsanto in America, and several other companies, and thus not theirs to give to anybody without permission. Outside consultants analyzing the intellectual property circumstances of Golden Rice painted a pessimistic picture; to get the project to the desired goal would require cutting through a thicket of intellectual property entanglements. The consultants uncovered some 70 patents, owned by 32 different companies and universities, embedded in Golden Rice (that number was an overestimate for countries in the developing world, where patents are not filed if they are considered unlikely to be useful there).

It was not clear how the original goal of Potrykus and Beyer could be achieved, given its complicated intellectual property circumstances and remaining technological challenges. Frustrated by unhelpful outside advice and the analysis of the patent situation, Potrykus and Beyer sought help from the agribusiness Zeneca, which merged with Novartis in 2000 to become Syngenta. It was one of the few companies with expertise in carotenoid production in plants, and in 2001 Potrykus and Beyer entered into a collaboration with it. Within a few years, scientists at Syngenta developed an improved version of Golden Rice, "SGR1" (Syngenta Golden Rice 1), which contained a higher level of beta-carotene. In 2005, they created a second improvement, GR2, which contains about 23 times as much beta-carotene as the original proof-of-concept Golden Rice. GR2 appears to contains enough beta-carotene to supply a large fraction of the RDA for people eating normal portions of it (168). In the new version of Golden Rice, the daffodil gene was replaced by the same gene taken from corn.

Complex negotiations began, orchestrated by Dr. Adrian Dubock, a scientist at Syngenta with experience in patents, product development, regulations, and humanitarian applications of biotechnology. These negotiations, between the inventors, Syngenta, Monsanto, and other patent holders, were successful. The development and free distribution of GR2 required the granting of patent rights by six key commercial entities. The outcome was an agreement in which Syngenta would have commercial development rights for GR2, but it would be licensed free of charge through the inventors (Potrykus and Beyer) for non-commercial use in the developing world. In addition, Dubock organized a new entity, the Golden Rice Humanitarian Board (GRHB), which would grant licenses and oversee the distribution of Golden Rice to agricultural research centres in those countries. The GRHB is presently supported by HarvestPlus (the organization behind much of the orange sweet potato developments in sub-Saharan Africa), the Gates Foundation, the World Bank, the Swiss Development and Collaboration Agency, USAID, the Syngenta Foundation, the Rockefeller Foundation, and the IRRI. Dubock has been the GRHB's project manager for Golden Rice since 2008 and the Executive Secretary of the organization since 2010. Amongst its members, GRHB includes Potrykus, Beyer, and Dubock, as well as Gary Toenniessen of the Rockefeller Foundation, who had organized the first meeting that considered a GE source of beta-carotene, and representatives of several national crop-breeding programs. Although the inventors were not initially pleased that they had had to turn to the agribusiness Syngenta to realize their goal, in 2010 Potrykus observed: "Without him [Adrian Dubock], the project would have ended already" (169).

The negotiated arrangement with Syngenta gave that company control over the use and sale of Golden Rice for commercial purposes. However, this was essentially a nonperforming asset; the company realized early on that there would not be a commercial market in North America and Europe, given the widespread opposition to Golden Rice as a GE product in the developed world, and the fact that vitamin A deficiency is not a significant problem there. In any case, people in developed countries do not eat enough rice to make much of a difference to their vitamin A status. The uncompensated contributions of Syngenta to the non-commercial development of Golden Rice included essential technology for the generation of improved lines of Golden Rice, continuing technical support, and the transfer of patent rights required for its distribution.

Although Golden Rice will not be a commercial success, in the developing world it has great potential as a remedy for vitamin A deficiency. In the arrangements between the GRHB and national agricultural research centres, no fees are levied, either by the GRHB or by Syngenta. When the technology reaches individual farmers, they will receive it free, and they will have the right to plant, harvest, save seed, and sell GR2, provided that their income is below $10,000 a year, which includes 99% of them. This agreement, and the actions of Syngenta and other patent holders, solved some major problems, but others remain.

Barriers to the development of Golden Rice as a source of vitamin A

Golden Rice was first patented in 1999, and the high-yield GR2 variety was produced in 2005 (168). But more than 10 years after the invention of GR2, the development of Golden Rice is still incomplete. The products needed (there will be several, differing for the various countries of intended use) must have growth qualities at least as good as the strains of rice currently grown. Farmers may like the idea of a healthier food for them and their children, but if that comes at the price of lower yield, they cannot afford to switch to it (the same issue had to be considered in the introduction of orange sweet potatoes in sub-Saharan Africa). It hasn't helped that its developers have recently had to switch to a different lead product due to problems of "yield drag." Crossing the Golden Rice trait into existing varieties of rice grown in different regions will require further field work and testing. Each round of hybridization takes a full growth cycle and must be carried out in biologically contained enclosures, even though Golden Rice has never been designated biohazardous by any scientific regulatory agency. The hybrid rice that results must be of at least as high quality agronomically as the rice grown previously, and also safe and effective at delivering vitamin A. As of the end of 2016, this has not yet been achieved for any GR2 hybrid rice.

The requirement for biohazard containment is partially responsible for the slow pace of development of Golden Rice. This requirement stems from an agreement signed in 2000, which became effective in 2003, called the Cartagena Protocol on Biosafety. Its 170 signatory countries agreed to use the "precautionary principle" in all biotechnological developments within their borders. It focuses on risks, even ones that are only imagined or highly unlikely. Different countries interpret the Cartagena Protocol differently. The efforts to cross the Golden Rice trait into indigenous strains of rice in India are seriously slowed down because the government dictates that such work must be carried out in an entirely enclosed, inconvenient construct called a Phytotron, which makes the job of the classical plant breeder almost impossible (170). In the Philippines, containment is considered to require a moat around Golden Rice fields, with rows of non-GE plants to catch any stray pollen. In the United States, which did not sign the Cartagena Protocol, GE crops are merely surrounded by a couple of rows of "pollen trap" non-GE plants. The concerns that led to the Cartagena Protocol stem from the beginnings of DNA cloning in bacteria, in the 1970s, when potential biohazards were not well understood. People involved in the development of Golden Rice feel that the early concerns have been answered, and that it is time to reconsider the issue of biosafety and reduce the encumbrances imposed by the Cartagena Protocol (170).

The efficacy of Golden Rice in delivering vitamin A through the diet is not yet fully established, although the testing that has been done indicates that it is apparently effective. A sample of GR2 was tested in the United States in 2009 (171). Five adults were given Golden Rice, and its conversion to vitamin A in their blood was determined. The ratio of conversion observed was 3.8:1 (it took 3.8 molecules of beta-carotene in Golden Rice to deliver one molecule of retinol in the blood), which was higher than anticipated. A second test was carried out, this time on Chinese school children (with repercussions that I'll describe a bit later), and here the results were even better: Golden Rice was just as effective as beta-carotene given in oil, and more than three times as efficient as spinach in delivering retinol to the children. At the rate observed, it would require only 100–150 grams of cooked Golden Rice to provide 60% of the RDA for a child six to eight years old (87). As critics have pointed out, both the American adult test group and the Chinese school children had reasonably good diets, including fats. Beta-carotene depends on fat for absorption during digestion, and further testing is needed to determine whether Golden Rice can supply adequate vitamin A to people on poor, low-fat diets.

Even if Golden Rice effectively delivers vitamin A, there is no guarantee that people will switch to eating it; the colour may put them off, even if its taste is indistinguishable from white rice (which it should be). However, there are already coloured rices in the world, such as the Bhutan Red variety, which are consumed willingly where they are grown. In sub-Saharan Africa, farmers and their families have happily switched from white sweet potatoes to the orange-fleshed types. Maybe colour doesn't matter much.

The publication that described the test of Golden Rice in China appeared on August 8, 2012 (87). The results were encouraging, in that the beta-carotene of the Golden Rice was efficiently converted to vitamin A in the blood. This study followed the earlier test on American adults that showed similar positive results (171). No ill effects were experienced in either study. But three weeks after publication of the Chinese study, there was an uproar, as Greenpeace denounced this use of Chinese children as "guinea pigs of the American biotechnology industry."[31] The Chinese government quickly changed its opinion about the study it had previously approved; it looked for, and claimed to find, irregularities in the proto-

---

31 Opponents of testing of vitamin A supplements in the Philippines in 1986 also invoked the metaphor of children as guinea pigs.

cols. The investigators had taken great pains to satisfy both American and Chinese research standards. Safeguards were built in, and the application was reviewed and approved by the Institutional Review Boards of both Tufts University (the academic home of the study leader, Dr. Guanwen Tang, who was born in China and who had led the first test on the American subjects), and the Chinese Academy of Preventive Medicine. The protocols claimed to be missing were Chinese documents and resided in China; they could not be produced. Chinese clinicians involved in the study — who experienced both the Greenpeace-led hysteria and, in some cases, middle-of-the-night visits by police — were sanctioned, and some withdrew their support. Tufts University instituted a review. It had no concerns about the integrity of the study data, the accuracy of the results, or the safety of the children who were the research subjects. None of the criticisms of Greenpeace or the Chinese government were upheld by the Tufts review.

The crux of the opposition was the claim that the Chinese authorities did not know that Golden Rice came from GE plants, which is not credible. Nevertheless, on the (undocumented) basis that some paperwork in China was incomplete, the university requested that the journal withdraw the publication, which it did, and it sanctioned Dr. Tang by forbidding her from discussing her results at scientific meetings. It also suspended her research privileges. Nearing retirement age, and tired of the struggle, Dr. Tang closed her world-class nutrition laboratory. (The dispiriting details of this affair are fully discussed elsewhere [172].)

The discrediting of the study in Chinese schoolchildren is particularly unfortunate, since China, despite rapid economic development, still has hundreds of millions of poor, rice-consuming people. Chinese authorities have estimated that 50% of the rural population and 30% of the urban population suffer from vitamin A deficiency, with 9% of all children in the country severely affected (173). This situation has not been helped by the reduction in consumption of orange sweet potatoes as economic conditions improved (the same process occurs in sub-Saharan Africa, as described in the previous chapter).

In another example of opposition to the development of Golden Rice, a group of 300–400 farmers and anti-GE campaigners attacked a field trial of Golden Rice at IRRI in the Bicol region of the Philippines in 2013 (174). The protesters surprised and overwhelmed the workers and security people at the site, who had been expecting to discuss the campaigners' concerns, and proceeded to trash the field of Golden Rice. Although the vandals claimed to be local farmers, the field workers saw that the local farmers in the crowd took no part in the destruction; they stood back, respecting their traditional belief that destruction of a living crop brings bad luck. Those carrying out the destruction were mostly young men, some of them with covered faces, who had been bussed in the previous day.

In echoes of the opposition that stopped the first attempt to study the effects of vitamin A deficiency in 1986 in the Philippines, a spokesman for the communist organization Asian Peasant Coalition issued a statement that said, in part:

> The development and promotion of Golden Rice illustrates an imperialist plunder of Asian agriculture that monopolizes seeds, limits bio-diversity and lessens dietary diversification. . . We condemn the IRRI, and Syngenta, for raking huge profits while destroying agriculture. . . What we need is genuine agrarian reform to resolve hunger and malnutrition. Further, we call on our members across Asia to uproot all GM crops in their country, intensify campaign [sic] against GMOs and strongly oppose its commercialization. (175)

Although this incident was discouraging, officials at the IRRI felt that progress toward the eventual goal could continue, as there were other fields of Golden Rice under study.

The most enduring opposition to Golden Rice is based on values, not facts. In the Appendix, I address the most frequent arguments against its development and use. They are founded largely on undocumented claims; there is simply no evidence in the scientific literature to support them, and the case against the biotechnology companies (that they are making profits from Golden Rice at the expense of people living in the developing world) is simply wrong, as already described. Ethical considerations are often brought up, based on the principle that it is wrong to produce GE plants in the first place, and even more wrong to introduce them into developing-world cultures. Such a value system is closely adhered to by Greenpeace, an organization implacably opposed not just to Golden Rice but to any GE solution to nutritional problems. This frame of mind is also behind a decision by a high court in the Philippines regarding the testing of "*Bt talong*," a GE version of eggplant that expresses Bt toxin, a bacterial protein that kills certain insect pests (Bt corn, resistant to the corn borer, is the same type of GE plant). In its decision on a case brought by Greenpeace and others (Greenpeace never misses an opportunity), the court heard from an opponent of testing named Dr. Ben Malayang III. In the filed court document (176), he argued, in part:

> in the event that indeed this would turn out to be bad for, after all, the [T]itanic engineers thought that it will never sink, there is at least full public participation in the acceptance of the risks . . . beyond the confines of the farm and the agricultural sector there may be other people out there and other sectors of our economy and society whose lives and practices and cultures may be effected [sic] because certain insects are no longer there to give them the kind of fruits that they have wanted for their own religious rites or anything like that. I mean I am just imagining, so we need to go beyond that.

The judge decided: "The Court is inclined to concur with the submission of Dr. Malayang" (whatever the exact meaning of his confusing statement might be). In other words, no *Bt talong* is to be tested, since the insect population might conceivably suffer, and so might human cultural life. The fact that the Bt toxin is already being expressed, apparently safely, on more than 800,000 acres of Bt-containing corn in the Philippines (the acreage of eggplant is a small fraction of this) wasn't considered in the decision. Nor was the fact that, in the absence of a GE version of Bt toxin in the plant itself, the spraying of Bt toxin — involving massively more of the toxin than produced in the GE plant — is a common agricultural practice worldwide. (Bt is considered so safe that it is even sprayed on organic corn in the developed world.)

That decision by the Philippine court in 2012 was challenged in 2015 but upheld. It remains to be seen what the practical results will be of these decisions, but they are worrisome to those who hope to provide the Philippine people with a cheap, safe source of vitamin A in a main staple crop, rice.

On the other side of the ethical arguments are those who think that the chance to save lives, or at least to test whether Golden Rice can save lives, more than outweighs qualms about genetic engineering. An international group of some of the most prominent scientists in the world has called for an end to what they refer to as the irrational opposition to the development of Golden Rice (174). The basis for their plea is the evidence that a real health problem exists, that Golden Rice shows every indication of addressing the problem, and that no direct negative health effects of *any* GE plant have so far been found.

CHAPTER 7

What Next?

The conundrum of present programs to provide vitamin A

Vitamin A is essential for human life, and our bodies are unable to produce it. A person not getting enough vitamin A for an extended period, particularly a preschool-age child, will suffer a loss of vision, declining general health, and, if the deficit persists, death. This essential micronutrient can be provided dietarily as either preformed vitamin A (retinol and its ester forms, which are present in some animal sources of food) or the provitamin A carotenoids, principally beta-carotene, which are present in many plants.

Since the discovery of the fundamental importance of vitamin A to life itself in the early 1980s, supplementation programs have been mounted in the developing world. Capsules containing vitamin A dissolved in oil work well and cost little — the usual target is two high-dosage pills a year, each costing about two cents. But capsules are much more expensive to administer than to produce; estimates run between one and two dollars per pill. With 500 million capsules a year being distributed, the cost of programs is significant. So far it has mostly been paid by agencies of the developed world, although these agencies are encouraging some developing countries to begin to cover the costs from their own budgets.

There are several limitations to supplementation programs, beginning with the fact that they do not solve the underlying cause of the deficiency, which is poor diet; if the priorities of the organizations and governments providing the supplements should change, the programs could collapse. Also, too many difficult-to-reach people do not have their needs met, as demonstrated by the limits of capsule programs — after decades of effort, only around 70% coverage in at-risk countries. Furthermore, capsule programs provide a bolus of vitamin A, followed by a long period (six months or sometimes 12) during which the levels dwindle, which is not an ideal regimen; it is better to have a continuous supply in the diet. Studies in the Philippines have found that this kind of feast-and-famine exposure, although it has benefit, is not ideal, as it does not greatly reduce overall deficiencies in serum retinol levels, a standard measure of vitamin A sufficiency (177). It is therefore necessary to consider and encourage other methods for providing vitamin A; the orange sweet potato in sub-Saharan Africa is an example of a worthwhile, and growing, success. Golden Rice, when it reaches full development, may be another.

Public health actions are profoundly sensitive to national priorities. Vitamin A deficiency in some countries of the developing world is in a state of re-evaluation. More than 30 years have passed since its effects on the health and mortality of children in Indonesia were documented. Since then, supplementation programs in many countries have provided children and pregnant women with the vitamin. But some prominent health administrators today question the need for, or the efficacy of, these programs because of what they perceive as overall improvements in nutrition and health, and the difficulty of directly demonstrating the beneficial effects of capsule programs today (177). This is particularly so in India, where opposition has arisen for several reasons (139, 178), even though, in the opinions of some Indian experts, the need for vitamin A supplementation still clearly exists (143).

It is true that in some countries, the effects of vitamin A deficiency have diminished as general nutrition has improved. Events in the Philippines over the decades illustrate the importance of politics and policy. After the first results from Indonesia in the 1980s showed that vitamin A supplementation prevented childhood deaths, Alfred Sommer and his team proposed a follow-up study in the Philippines, to confirm the conclusion in another setting. As described already, that attempt was thwarted by anti-American sentiment. More recently, evident progress in reducing vitamin A deficiency in that country is being used as an argument against the need for Golden Rice, which is being developed most intensely at the IRRI in Manila. There has, indeed, been a significant reduction in vitamin A deficiency in a number of Asian countries, including the Philippines, where levels of vitamin A deficiency in children below the age of five went from around 40% in 2003 to 15% by 2008 (179). The WHO now lists the public health challenge posed by vitamin A deficiency in that country as "mild." The levels of evident deficiency in Southeast and East Asian countries overall has also declined, according to one recent study (180). But vitamin A deficiency remains an important issue, particularly in South Asia, China, and sub-Saharan Africa.

The decline in vitamin A deficiency in the Philippines is unsurprising, since vitamin A supplementation programs using capsules have existed there for more than 20 years. According to the Food and Nutrition Research Institute of the Philippines, 92% of children under age five in the Philippines are currently reached by twice-a-year vitamin A capsule programs (181). In addition, general nutrition has improved. The experience in that country over the years reflects patterns elsewhere, with vitamin A sufficiency in part reflecting better nutrition, which improves with economic conditions.

But many children still suffer nightblindness and have low blood retinol levels, as assessed by the WHO. Vitamin A deficiency still affects more than 1.7 million children under five in the Philippines, and 500,000 pregnant and nursing women. Vitamin A deficiency is an even greater problem in India and China. Because it is not ethically acceptable to carry out further, definitive tests of the effects of vitamin A deficiency (it would be unethical to deprive children of vitamin A in order to compare them to a peer group receiving the vitamin, knowing what we know), the proof that vitamin A supplementation helps must be taken from the older data and by indirect tests such as serum retinol levels.

This is the conundrum of vitamin A supplementation: as capsule delivery programs take hold, and as general conditions improve, visual and other health problems of children decline, suggesting to some that no further action is required. Yet even in countries where it has had a beneficial effect but where nutritional needs are not fully met, the need for supplementation continues. If capsule delivery programs stop today, there will undoubtedly be a rise in nightblindness and children's death rates tomorrow. And to drive the rates of children's medical problems even lower requires a complementary program for providing vitamin A. At the moment, the only program that looks like it might succeed in the rice-dependent world is Golden Rice.

Beyond preventing nightblindness and death

Nightblindness was the first symptom intensively studied as a marker of vitamin A deficiency. In turn, it was found to be a correlate of childhood death, often due to infection. But besides the incidence of nightblindness and premature death, and criteria such as retinol levels, there are other health concerns regarding vitamin A sufficiency. They stem from research on laboratory animals. In the early stages of vitamin discovery, experiments with rats, mice and dogs played a large role, as described in earlier chapters. These included: the morbidity and mortality studies on rats by the pioneers Hopkins and McCollum, which showed stunted growth, among other effects; the blindness studied in rats by Dowling and Wald; and the role of retinoic acid in gene regulation in animals. All of these effects are demonstrably similar or identical in humans. Therefore, it is worrisome that animal research shows that vitamin A deficiency poses a significant risk, beyond blindness and mortality, to the health of the newborn and young. In one study, oral tolerance to antigens (a measure of the risk of allergy) was inhibited in neonatal mice by vitamin A deficiency (53). At the other end of the immunological response spectrum, vitamin A deficiency impairs both antibody and cellular immune reactions to antigens (47, 54). Vitamin A deficiency was found to cause a loss of beta cells in the pancreas — the origin of insulin and the insulin response — and, as expected, this was accompanied by hyperglycaemia (elevated blood sugar) (55). In another study, rats deprived of vitamin A delivered pups with multiple birth defects (39, 56). Given the historical parallels between vitamin effects in humans and laboratory animals, it would be irresponsible to think that these results are of no concern for human health, particularly of newborns and young children, because they indicate that the health effects of vitamin A insufficiency are not limited to visual problems, sensitivity to infection, and premature death.

Challenges to rational approaches to vitamin A deficiency

Its proponents believe that Golden Rice could significantly reduce vitamin A deficiency in rice-growing countries, even where capsule distribution already exists. But there is a great deal of opposition to GE foods, particularly in developed countries. This surely stems in part from a general loss of trust in science. An example of this mistrust was described in a recent article in *The Globe and Mail*. After the nuclear disaster at the Fukushima reactor in Japan, people living on the west coast of North America became concerned about the possible arrival of radioactive debris from across the Pacific. This was not unreasonable. To determine whether that was actually happening, some scientists set up monitoring sites on the northwest Pacific coast in British Columbia. A former colleague of mine at the University of Victoria has been assessing the radioactivity washing up on our shores and incorporated into our fish since 2014. His results show no indication of contamination from the Fukushima nuclear reactor. The news article (November 1, 2015) described the abuse being directed at him because he reported this finding. He has been called a "shill" for the nuclear energy industry and a "sham scientist," neither of which is true. I know him to be a careful, smart, and productive young scientist, a member of a first-rate academic unit. He has no connections to any industry, let alone nuclear energy.

The vituperative and often hate-filled reactions to the ocean-monitoring program are irrational and don't represent most people's opinions. Still, only 40% of Americans apparently have "a great deal of confidence" in the scientific community. Medicine also fares poorly: between 1974 and 2012, those having "a great deal of confidence" in medicine declined from 61% to 39% (182). The issue of GE foods falls within the worlds of both science and medicine. The degree of trust in authorities in these areas is apparently declining, at least in the United States. And mistrust in general appears to be growing: only 19% of millenials, people between the ages of 16 and 36 in 2016, say they feel that most people can be trusted, compared to 40% of the "boomer" generation, according to a recent column by David Brooks in *The New York Times*.

There is some basis for a sceptical view of science, particularly in relation to medicine and health. What are people to make of issues such as the supposed link between dietary fat and heart disease, first proposed by medical authorities in the early 1960s and then relentlessly promoted by establishment health agencies? Evidence for such a link for the vast majority of the population does not exist and never did (183). It was a "just so story" made up by supposedly sound medical and scientific authorities who have now changed their collective mind.[32] It made sense to them (eat fat, get fat), so they took it too far and put it out as scientific fact. And then there are the recent analyses questioning the reliability of research, particularly in medicine and human health, which is the kind of research that matters most to the majority of people. Complex areas, such as psychology (184), and drug testing in cancer treatment (185), are particularly vulnerable to irreproducibility. There are nuanced arguments about what such irreproducibility actually signifies, and just how true it is, particularly in the "harder" sciences, where numbers and chemical structures dominate. But still, it's being widely talked and written about. It's also damaging to rational thinking when a supposed medical authority presents data showing that autism is linked to vaccination for common childhood diseases. The fact that this "medical authority," a physician named Andrew Wakefield, was posting fake data hasn't erased that connection for many people; his work was published in one of the most highly regarded medical journals (*The Lancet*). Nor did it help when his perfidy was uncovered not by his peers, the way it's supposed to happen, but by a smart and persistent journalist.

---

32 A term sometimes used to describe fantasized scientific narratives is "just so stories," after the title of the book of fables collected by Rudyard Kipling.

Adding to the problem is the sensationalized over-interpretation of some scientific news, particularly having to do with medicine and nutrition, in the popular press. Fear, one of the most saleable products of modern media, is constantly invoked in stories about dangerous health effects caused by, for example, eating bacon. That's not to deny that processed meats contain some ingredients that increase the odds of diseases such as cancer. Yet this information was recently presented as frightening percentage increases in cancer deaths from what amounts to excessive consumption (e.g., that the risk of colorectal cancer increases by 21% if you eat lots of bacon three times a day), rather than that the annual diagnoses of colorectal cancer even for typical bacon eaters is increased by one case per 10,000 people, and the increase in deaths, one in 30,000.[33] The Physicians Committee for Responsible Medicine, just one of the professional information platforms available to a concerned public, dourly notes, "No amount of processed meat is considered safe for consumption." On the other side of the coin, we find news stories bursting with unjustified optimism that a particular research discovery will, usually within five years, result in significant improvements in our lives; such reports are often followed by. . . silence. Neither fear nor unrealistic expectation helps develop rational ideas about science and technology.

Also, thanks to the Internet, we are living in an age of facile "wisdom" and personal-choice "facts." Support can be found online for almost any position, mainstream or contrarian. Surprisingly, perhaps, some of the highest levels of scepticism toward conventional science and technology reside in communities with the highest levels of educational and socioeconomic achievement. Marin County, across the Golden Gate Bridge from San Francisco, has been featured in the news as a hotbed of opposition to vaccination against childhood diseases such as whooping cough and measles. It's no wonder that this opposition carries weight — its proponents are Very Serious People, to use a pejorative favoured by the economist Paul Krugman. For years, many parents in Marin refused to have their

---

33 Many of those stories are, as Yogi Berra would have said, déjà vu all over again. I remember teaching medical students about the cancer potential of nitrates and nitrites used in curing meats 35 years ago.

children vaccinated against childhood diseases. Fortunately, that opposition has recently begun to diminish.

In a poll by the PEW Research Center published in 2015, the consensus among American scientists that GE organisms are safe stands at 88% (186). Yet 57% of the general public in America say GE foods are unsafe, and 67% do not believe that scientists understand the science behind GMOs. As another indication of what scientists think, a report in 2010 from the European Commission Directorate-General for Research and Innovations also concluded that GE plants are safe (187).

This is consistent with the position of many of the most prominent scientific bodies in the world, including the US National Academy of Sciences, the American Medical Association, and the WHO. Despite scientists overwhelmingly thinking that Golden Rice poses no biohazard, many people and organizations argue strenuously that it does. Foremost among them is Greenpeace, whose opposition is exemplified by what happened in the study involving Chinese schoolchildren who were fed Golden Rice, as described in Chapter 6. In June of 2016, 110 Nobel Prize laureates, mostly from the sciences but also winners of Economics, Literature, and Peace Prizes, begged Greenpeace to stop "bashing" GMOs in general and Golden Rice in particular (188).

Viewed objectively, there clearly are reasons to pursue the development and testing of Golden Rice, and other promising products of GE food research; people's health and lives are at stake. It is painless to unequivocally oppose all such initiatives when your own food supply is replete with micronutrients, including vitamin A. The issue looks different when children are going blind and dying because of a lack of it, as they are in many parts of the world where there is no other solution.

We are wise to be cautious — but not to the point of immobility on a critical nutritional issue. New technologies should be examined for benefit and risk, and an informed decision made about their deployments. For example, Bt corn (corn genetically engineered to express the bacterial-derived Bt toxin) is effective and safe for mammals, including humans, because the toxin is active only at the neutral pH of the gut of the corn borer, which it targets and kills, compared to the acidic pH of our guts. For decades before Bt corn was invented, Bt toxin was sprayed directly onto crops; this continues today, and its residual presence is deemed acceptable even on organic corn. Genetically engineered Bt corn obviates the need for spraying and is more effective. There is little objective argument against its use, and its benefit-to-risk ratio is high. On the other hand, the heavy use of Roundup-Ready crops — GE plants into which a gene has been introduced that makes them resistant to the herbicide glyphosate (Roundup) — has produced significant problems because it has resulted in Roundup-resistant "superweeds."[34] This problem bears some similarity to the overuse of antibiotics, which has led to a rise in antibiotic-resistant disease-causing bacteria. Evolution never sleeps, and the occurrence of a mutated, resistant form will give the organism a selective advantage. Continuing analysis of the risks (increasing) and benefits (stationary or decreasing) of using Roundup-resistant crops is necessary.

Some nuances of genetic engineering

There are detailed analyses of the subject of GE food in two particularly readable and authoritative books on food and nutrition: *Just Food*, by James E. McWilliams (189), and *Mendel in the Kitchen*, by Nina Fedoroff and Marie Brown (190). On balance, and after listing all of the facts and examining them carefully, these writers conclude that, with care, the introduction of GE technology into agriculture is effectively an extension of the development of agricultural practices that began 10,000 years ago with the taming of wild grasses. GE plants are another round in the endless struggle to produce more and better food with fewer resources. It began with the hybridization and selection of cereal crops and milk-producing animals. Such genetic modification, involving human-controlled evolution and selection, is generally accepted, even when it results in significant genetic changes. Carefully controlled, the use of modern genetic technology to achieve similar goals should be just as acceptable. Rational analysis leads to the conclusion that it's not the technology that matters,

---

34 "Superweeds" that are resistant to Roundup are the result of mutations in the weed's genome; they are not due to migration of the resistance gene into the weed's genome. In other words, the source of the problem is the (over)use of glyphosate, not GE technology.

it's the results of that technology that are significant. It would be ironic if heavy doses of irradiation or chemicals — as are sometimes used to produce mutated plant variants by conventional genetics, and which profoundly mess up genomes — should be allowed but not GE methods, which in the case of Golden Rice result in the addition of three genes into the background of 20,000 or so and produce a genome with a precisely known sequence.

McWilliams (189) also raises a different point in *Just Food*. He believes that

> a more rational approach to genetic modification technology would be to support its application to essential food crops in developing countries . . . Flood-tolerant rice, drought-tolerant sweet potatoes, salt-tolerant cassava . . . As it now stands, we're mired in a situation in which agribusiness employs biotechnology to grow staple commodities to feed cows (and cars) while advocates of agroecology and organic methods battle what they call Frankenfoods . . . "the way forward lies in harnessing the power of modern technology, but harnessing it wisely in the interest of the poor and hungry and with respect for the environment." (p. 216; the passage McWilliams quotes is from agricultural ecologist Sir Gordon Conway)

Rational as this approach is, critics of GE crops turn it into an indictment when they claim that the wealthy countries are using the developing world as a laboratory, with its human populations as guinea pigs. Proponents of such a position are not swayed by the evidence, since they distrust the scientific approach. But what should be a serious counterargument for anyone interested in helping vitamin A-deficient people in the developing world is the breathtaking developed-world paternalism embodied in unequivocal opposition to using GE to save the vision, the general health, and the very lives of children. As quoted evidence in the Appendix indicates, developing countries have largely embraced the results of GE agriculture when it helps them. Is it really ethical for critics in developed nations to forbid the full benefit of GE foods if those are found to be effective and safe?

A major concern often cited by critics of GE agriculture is the expansion of monocrops — the growing of one type of crop, with one type of seed, over huge tracts of land. This can have serious effects on both biodiversity and the spread of disease. But there is no direct connection between monocropping and the use of GE crops such as Golden Rice; those issues must be addressed separately. The foundational Golden Rice must be crossed into whatever rice variety is being grown in a particular region before it becomes a practical alternative. The degree of "monocropping" before and after the introduction of the Golden Rice trait will be the same. The rice growers who feed three billion people in the developing world practice monocropping on a large scale already, out of necessity. In the end, we need to adopt best practices, however they originate.

The successful application of genetics to medicine, either already achieved or predicted, strikes most people as beneficial, a payback for the billions spent on basic research. Production of insulin from recombinant DNA in bacteria or yeast is one such example. Synthesis of monoclonal antibodies[35] for the detection and treatment of certain types of cancer is another. On the other hand, the application of molecular genetics to the food-production industry leaves many people wary, or even opposed. The modern world is one that encourages curiosity, development, and application, and it is difficult to see how we could pursue, for example, the use of genetic techniques to find a cure for cancer but at the same time be prevented from looking at the development of GE agriculture, even if we wanted to. But regulation of practical outcomes *can* be imposed, to insure that the products of science do not add to societal problems. It is possible to stop or regulate the application of a genetic technology that is found to be harmful, even if the basic knowledge to produce it is in the public domain. An example is forbidding the use of Bovine Growth Hormone (produced from recombinant DNA) to increase milk production, as has been done in most advanced countries because of its deleterious health effects on cattle (the United States is an exception). Roundup-Ready crops may

35 Monoclonal antibodies have figured prominently in the news over the past decade. They are antibodies (immunoglobulin molecules) created in the laboratory and then cloned that are selected for their ability to recognize specific targets, including bacteria, viruses, and cancer cells.

soon be facing regulation, as resistance to glyphosate spreads ever more widely. Such control would be parallel to the regulation of antibiotics in the cattle feeding industry, a desperately needed development that is slowly coming into being. Suppression of discovery and invention is almost impossible in a free society, but regulation of the use of the products of those processes is not.

There have been three seething genetic controversies over the past 100 years. The first was eugenics. Although it had its origins in the work of Darwin's half-cousin Francis Galton, it came to its apogee during the period 1920 to 1945. It was largely focused on human mental and physical capacities as determined by genetics, leading to the passage of forced sterilization laws in several countries, the last of which were not repealed until the 1970s. In contrast to the two later controversies, this really did, in part, involve an evil genetic practice. Some major scientific figures became entangled in eugenics, even though their interest was usually scientific and did not include forced intervention in human affairs. The spectre of eugenics applied as a "solution" to human problems still lurks in the background. (The issues are again coming to the fore in light of new developments in editing the DNA of living cells, which suggest that we may soon be in a position, technically if not morally, to "improve" humans.)

The second public issue involving genetics erupted in the 1970s, when many people felt that the cloning of DNA was a threat to human well-being and the biological world more generally. Scientists were initially uncertain about the level of threat, although many non-scientists had no such doubts — the city council of Cambridge, Massachusetts, behind its mayor, Al Velucci, forbade the study of recombinant DNA in that city in 1976, although the ban was lifted after just seven months. With the creation of guidelines, and the accumulation of evidence showing a lack of danger associated with the cloning of DNA, public opposition gradually died down. This has not prevented the imposition of the Cartagena Protocol, largely arising from those earlier concerns, to the development and testing of GE foods, even though most of the issues giving rise to it have long been resolved.

The third controversy related to genetics is in full flower today and is associated with genetic engineering, especially of food plants. There is no doubt that caution should be exercised in any new technology, and that the agenda should not be handed over to a commercial entity whose primary motivation is to make a profit for its shareholders. But nor should we refuse to examine that technology to see whether it can improve conditions for humanity, particularly in less developed parts of the world. There are excellent descriptions of the issues related to genetic engineering in the books by Fedoroff and Brown, and by McWilliams. There needs to be an enlightened discussion and educated decision-making. In the end, science and scientists who understand it must be included in that discussion.

Part of the power of science is that some questions can be answered; in such cases, a controversy or disagreement can eventually be resolved, and the proponents of the incorrect side of the argument will stop talking. In this sense, science enjoys a great intellectual luxury, since most issues in the world don't lend themselves to binary resolution. The latter includes opposition to Golden Rice, which is now almost entirely about values, not science. The scientific arguments are always brought up, but they have been answered (see the Appendix). But no amount of scientific evidence can change the mind of someone who believes that GE categorically should never be used to solve nutritional problems.

Rational decisions about genetically engineered foods such as Golden Rice should be made according to each particular case and its context. The teasing apart of these issues, the weighing of evidence, and the testing of possibilities require an unprejudiced analytical approach, an ability to interpret evidence, as well as sensitivity to cultural contexts. Whether that will happen in the near future, to the degree it should, is not clear. There is a great deal of biased advocacy in the world, and the challenge is to replace it with a clear and evidence-based approach. Discourse is important, but it must be based on facts, not on just so stories.

APPENDIX

Objections to Golden Rice and GE Foods

Where an association of quoted authors with the biotechnology industry may be relevant, their affiliations are provided. A number of the issues are discussed more fully in the text.

OBJECTION TO GE	EXAMINATION OF THE ISSUE
GE foods contain novel allergens and toxins and are dangerous to human health.	Several thousand peer-reviewed reports have demonstrated the safety of GE foods. None has identified any hazard to the health of humans or other animals.[36] Golden Rice has shown no harm to date but requires further testing, which is being vigorously resisted by opponents of GE.
Golden Rice is a mechanism for agribusiness to profit off the backs of farmers in the developing world and make them beholden to the industry in the future.	Golden Rice has been given to the GRHB to distribute freely. Any farmer making less than $10,000 per year will not have to pay anything and can use his/her own harvested rice as seed.

36 See A. Nicolia, A. Manzo, F. Veronesi, and D. Rosellini (2013), An overview of the last 10 years of genetically engineered crop safety research. *Critical Reviews in Biotechnology* 34(1): 77-88. The authors are from the University of Perugia, Italy, and the Italian Ministry of Agriculture, Food and Forestry. A different kind of analysis is reported by R. E. Goodman and J. Wise of the University of Nebraska, Study Number BIO-02-2006, which can be found online at http://www.allergenonline.org/Golden%20 Rice%202%20Bioinformatics%20FARRP%202006.pdf. In that study, three exhaustive, computationally based searches were made for known allergenic protein segments in the three proteins introduced into Golden Rice. None were found. These authors list some research support from industry.

Golden Rice will be a monoculture and will drive out other crops.	The populations for whom Golden Rice is developed already consume rice as their major, monocultured nutrient. Crossing the "Golden" trait into local varieties of rice doesn't change the degree of monocropping.
There are many other, cheaper solutions to vitamin A deficiency, such as balanced diets.	There aren't. Balanced diets are certainly the best solution but are simply not affordable for most people who live in vitamin A-deficient areas.
100 million dollars have already been spent developing Golden Rice, yet it still isn't available. Use the money for things that work.	The current cost of vitamin A capsule programs is over 500 million dollars a year. If Golden Rice can be brought into production, it will be almost free.
Golden Rice is a "Trojan horse" for industry to get other GE products into the fields and markets of the world.	There are already 200 million hectares (almost 500 million acres) of GE crops, most of them in the developing world, which has largely embraced them. No Trojan horses are required.
All GE is bad.	Some is good, some is damaging, some is unnecessary. A recent analysis shows that the use of GE crops has, overall, reduced chemical pesticide use by 37%, increased crop yields by 22%, and increased farmers' profits by 68%, mostly in the developing world (191).[37]

---

37 The authors of this study are in the Department of Agricultural Economics and Rural Development at Georg-August University, in Goettingen, Germany, and declare no competing interest.

Although rice mostly self-pollinates (the same plant produces the pollen and is fertilized by it), the incidence of cross-pollination is not zero. The "Golden" trait may contaminate other types of domesticated or wild rice.	Any transfer of the "Golden" trait would be readily visible. Also, it has no intrinsic growth advantage, so it will not have a selective advantage in any accidental outcross. Finally, many green-leafed plants already have the enzymes required to produce beta-carotene.
According to the Greenpeace website, "It is irresponsible to impose Golden Rice on people if it goes against their religious beliefs, cultural heritage and sense of identity, or simply because they do not want it."	True. But there's no obvious way to force someone who doesn't wish to grow it to do so. The developing world has voluntarily adopted other GE crops because of their advantages.
The introduction of Golden Rice will play havoc with export markets.	There would be no reason for a large-scale grower (the only kind that would want to export rice) to use Golden Rice, which is intended for local use.
Human DNA will be contaminated by DNA for the GR trait.	Some DNA from food may enter our cells — the evidence is not settled. But the genes for the Golden Rice trait are "natural" and found in all foods that make beta-carotene, so we're already exposed to them.

From an anti-GMO website: "Research from Canada (the first of its kind) has successfully identified the presence of pesticides associated with genetically modified foods in maternal, fetal and non-pregnant women's blood [citing (192)]. They also found the presence of Monsanto's Bt toxin."	This research has been discredited by a number of scientific studies.[38] In any case, it is irrelevant to Golden Rice, in which no pesticide is involved.
Gluten disorders have been linked to GE.	There is no peer-reviewed publication that backs such claims, which are based on press releases, anecdotes, or unre-viewed publications.
Roundup (glyphosate) and Roundup-Ready maize cause rats to die earlier (193).	This work has been comprehensively dis-credited and has been withdrawn from the peer-reviewed journal of original publication (it was subsequently pub-lished without peer review). In any case, the Golden Rice trait has nothing to do with Roundup resistance or use.

38 See, for example, U. Mueller and J. Gorst (2012), Comment on "Maternal and fetal exposure to pesticides associated to genetically modified foods in Eastern Townships of Quebec, Canada" by A. Aris and S. Leblanc. *Reproductive Toxicology* 33(3): 401-402. The authors are from Food Standards, Australia and New Zealand.

GLOSSARY

amine — a chemical with an amino group ($-NH_2$); organic compounds that are derivatives of ammonia (NH_3).

beriberi — a neurological disease due to a deficiency of vitamin B1 (thiamin); characterized by loss of feeling in the limbs, paralysis of wrists and feet, wasting of muscles, weakness, heart enlargement, and heart failure.

beta-carotene — a retinoid found in carrots, orange sweet potatoes, dark green leafy vegetables, and other plants, which can be converted to retinal (functional vitamin A) in the human body; beta-carotene and other retinoids are referred to as "provitamin A."

Bitot's spots — raised, foamy or pearly-appearing patches on the conjunctiva of the eye, due to deposits of an insoluble protein, keratin; an early stage of deterioration of the eye due to vitamin A deficiency, which overall is referred to as xerophthalmia (see below).

bran — the outer coat of a cereal grain, rich in B vitamins such as thiamin.

calorie — a measure of the energy content of a food.

carbohydrate — a group of foods that contain sugars or starches (sugars and starches are essentially similar in nutritional value).

conjunctiva — the mucous membrane that lines the inner surfaces of the eyelids and the exposed surface of the eyeball.

epidemiology — the study of the patterns, causes, and control of disease in a population.

fat — foods that are made up of esters of fatty acids and glycerol, as well as other compounds with similar solubility properties, such as steroids; also called lipids.

GE — genetic engineering; altering the genetics of an organism in a pre-dicted way by the directed manipulating of its genomic DNA; the product is one form of GMO (genetically modified organism).

GMO — genetically modified organism, which can include modification by mutagenesis with chemicals or radiation, genetic engineering, or even conventional plant breeding.

GRHB — the Golden Rice Humanitarian Board, the organization charged with distributing licenses to use Golden Rice to national agricultural agencies in the developing world, for further develop-ment and then distribution to farmers in those countries. Licenses issued by the GRHB for using Golden Rice are free.

hypervitaminosis A — an excess of vitamin A.

IRRI — International Rice Research Institute, located in Manila, Philippines.

IU — International Unit, an amount of a vitamin (or other biological material) as defined by its activity; one IU of (preformed) vitamin A corresponds to 0.3 micrograms of pure retinol.

keratomalacia — a late stage of deterioration of the eye as a result of vita-min A deficiency, in which there is extensive ulceration and tissue death in the cornea, leading to blindness. The overall process of deterioration is referred to as xerophthalmia (see below).

macronutrients — the major calorie contributors in food, comprising pri-marily carbohydrates, fats, and proteins.

micronutrients — essential nutrients that are required in small amounts, including minerals and vitamins.

mineral — a non-organic micronutrient, such as zinc, iron, calcium, po-tassium, or sodium, required for animal nutrition.

morbidity — illness or a diseased state.

mortality — death.

nightblindness — the loss of vision in low light, due to a decreased function of the rod cells of the eye, often caused by a deficiency in vitamin A, which provides the essential visual chromophore (retinal) of these cells.

pellagra — a life-threatening disease caused by a deficiency of niacin (vitamin B3) in the diet; symptoms include inflammation of the skin, diarrhoea and mental disturbances.

preformed vitamin A — a group of compounds, including retinol, retinal, and retinoic acid, which are responsible for vitamin A effects in the human body. Preformed vitamin A is the directly active form of the vitamin.

protein — a group of chemicals consisting of long chains of amino acids and comprising an important macronutrient.

provitamin A — a group of compounds that can be converted to preformed vitamin A, found in plants such as spinach, carrots, and other deep green or orange vegetables and fruits. The most prominent provitamin A is beta-carotene.

RDA — recommended daily allowance (also "recommended dietary allowance"; in this book, it refers to "daily"); the daily intake, usually of a micronutrient such as a vitamin, that is recommended by national nutritional agencies.

retinal — the aldehyde form of vitamin A, which is the form in which it functions in the visual system of animals; retinal is oxidized retinol.

retinoic acid — the acid form of vitamin A, which corresponds to oxidized retinal; retinoic acid functions in the regulation of various genes but not in the visual process.

retinol — the alcohol form of vitamin A, which is also a common form found in foods derived from animal sources and in vitamin supplements.

retinyl esters — retinol that is conjugated to a fatty acid, such as retinyl palmitate, which is an ester of retinol and the fatty acid palmitate, a normal dietary constituent.

rhodopsin — a light-sensitive, retinal-containing pigment in the rod cells of the retina of the eye, necessary to convert light into a nerve signal. Rod cells are responsive to low light levels.

rickets — a disease caused by a deficiency of vitamin D, characterized by poor bone development and impaired growth.

thiamin — a B-complex vitamin (vitamin B1) found in whole grains and other foods such as nuts and legumes, as well as the bran of grains such as rice.

vitamin A — the group of compounds comprising preformed vitamin A and provitamin A.

vitamin B group — the group of vitamins, including thiamin and niacin, that are often referred to as "water soluble," although some are not; all are essential for normal functioning of the body, but some are so ubiquitous that deficiency seldom occurs.

vitamin C — a water-soluble vitamin, a deficiency of which leads to scurvy.

vitamin D — a fat-soluble vitamin found in fish, especially the livers, and in eggs as well as other foods; it is also produced in the skin by irradiation with UV light such as is present in sunlight.

WHO — World Health Organization (a branch of the United Nations).

xerophthalmia — the symptoms of visual deterioration that can be due to deficiency in vitamin A; begins with nightblindness, followed by the development of Bitot's spots, and ending with complete loss of vision due to damage to the cornea (this last stage is referred to as keratomalacia).

WORKS CITED

1. Sommer, A. 2013. *10 Lessons in Public Health.* The Johns Hopkins University Press, Baltimore.

2. World Health Organization. 2011. *Guideline: Vitamin A Supplementation in Infants and Children 6-59 Months of Age.* WHO, Geneva.

3. Kornberg, A. 1989. *For the Love of Enzymes. The Odyssey of a Biochemist.* Harvard University Press , Cambridge, MA.

4. McCay, C. M., M. F. Crowell, and L. A. Maynard. 1935. The Effect of Retarded Growth Upon the Length of Life Span and Upon the Ultimate Body Size. *J. Nutr.* 10:63-79.

5. Semba, R. D. 1999. Vitamin A as "Anti-Infective" Therapy, 1920-1940. *J. Nutr.* 129:783-791.

6. Eijkman, C. 1965. Nobel Prize in Physiology or Medicine, 1929: Antineuritic Vitamin and Beriberi. In *Nobel Lectures, Physiology or Medicine 1922-1941.* Elsevier, Amsterdam.

7. Hopkins, F. G. 1912. Feeding Experiments Illustrating the Importance of Accessory Factors in Normal Dietaries. *J. Physiol.* 44:425-460.

8. McCollum, E. V., and M. Davis. 1913. The Necessity of Certain Lipins in the Diet During Growth. *J. Biol. Chem.* 15:167-175.

9. Osborne, T., and L. B. Mendel. 1913. The Relation of Growth to the Chemical Constituents of the Diet. *J. Biol. Chem.* 15:311-326.

10. McCollum, E. V., and C. Kennedy. 1916. The Dietary Factors Operating in the Production of Polyneuritis. *J. Biol. Chem.* 24:491-502.

11. McCollum, E. V. 1964. *The Autobiography of Elmer Verner McCollum.* University of Kansas Press, Lawrence, Kansas.

12. McCollum, E. V., N. Simmonds, and H. T. Parsons. 1917. A Biological Analysis of Pellagra-Producing Diets. V. The Nature of the Dietary Deficiencies of a Diet Derived From Peas, Wheat Flour, and Cottonseed Oil. *J. Biol. Chem.* 33:411-423.

13. Semba, R. D. 2012. *The Vitamin A Story: Lifting the Shadow of Death.* Karger, Basel.

14. Hart, E. B. 1918. Professional Courtesy. *Science* 47:220-221.

15. Karrer, P. 1966. Carotenoids, Flavins and Vitamin A and B2. Nobel Lecture, 1937. In *Nobel Lectures, Chemistry 1922-1941*. Elsevier, Amsterdam.

16. Drummond, J. C. 1920. LIX. The Nomenclature of the So-called Accessory Food Factors (Vitamins). *Biochem. J.* 14:660.

17. Park, E. A. 1923. The Etiology of Rickets. *Physiol. Rev.* 3:106-163.

18. Carpenter, K. J., and L. Zhao. 1999. Forgotten Mysteries in the Early History of Vitamin D. *J. Nutr.* 129:923-927.

19. Wolf, G. 2004. The Discovery of Vitamin D: The Contribution of Adolf Windaus. *J. Nutr.* 134:1299-1302.

20. Chick, H., E. J. H. Dalyell, E. M. Hume, H. M. M. Mackay, and H. Henderson-Smith. 1922. The Aetiology of Rickets in Infants: Prophylactic and Curative Observations at the Vienna University Kinderklinik. *The Lancet* ii:7-11.

21. Carpenter, K. J. 2008. Harriette Chick and the Problem of Rickets. *J. Nutr.* 138:827-832.

22. McCollum, E. V., N. Simmonds, J. E. Becker, and P. G. Shipley. 1922. Studies on Experimental Rickets. XXI. An Experimental Demonstration of the Existence of a Vitamin which Promotes Calcium Deposition. *J. Biol. Chem.* 53:293-312.

23. Hume, E. G., and H. H. Smith. 1923. The Effect of Air, which Has Been Exposed to the Radiations of the Mercury-vapour Quartz Lamp, in Promoting the Growth of Rats, Fed on a Diet Deficient in Fat-Soluble Vitamins. *Biochem. J.* 17:364-372.

24. Steenbock, H., and A. Black. 1924. The Induction of Growth-promoting and Calcifying Properties in a Ration by Exposure to Ultra-violet Light. *J. Biol. Chem.* 61:405-422.

25. Bollet, A. J. 1992. Politics and Pellagra: The Epidemic of Pellagra in the U.S. in the Early Twentieth Century. *Yale Journal of Biology and Medicine* 65:211-221.

26. Szent-Gyorgy, A. 1928. CLXXIII. Observations on the Function of Peroxidase Systems and the Chemistry of the Adrenal Cortex. Description of a New Carbohydrate Derivative. *Biochem. J.* 22:1387-1409.

27. Svirbely, J. L., and C. G. King. 1931. The Preparation of Vitamin C Concentrates from Lemon Juice. *J. Biol. Chem.* 94:483-490.

28. King, C. G., and W. A. Waugh. 1932. The Chemical Nature of Vitamin C. *Science* 75:357-358.

29. Svirbely, J., and Szent-Gyorgyi. 1932. Hexuronic Acid as the Antiscorbutic Factor. *Nature* 129:576.

30. Hoffbrand, A. V., and D. G. Weir. 2001. Historical Review. The History of Folic Acid. *Brit. J. Haematol.* 113:579-589.

31. Roe, D. A. 1978. Lucy Wills (1888-1964): A Biographical Sketch. *J. Nutr.* 108:1379-1383.

32. Lobo, G. P., S. Hessel, A. Eichinger, N. Noy, A. R. Moise, A. Wyss, K. Palczewski, *et al.* 2010. ISX is a Retinoic Acid-sensitive Gatekeeper that Controls Intestinal β,β-carotene Absorption and Vitamin A Production. *FASEB J.* 24:1656-1666.

33. Novotny, J. A., D. J. Harrison, R. Pawlosky, V. P. Flanagan, E. H. Harrison, and A. C. Kurilich. 2010. Beta-carotene Conversion to Vitamin A Decreases as the Dietary Dose Increases in Humans. *J. Nutr.* 140:915-918.

34. Krinsky, N. I. 1989. Antioxidant Functions of Carotenoids. *Free Radical Biology and Medicine* 7:617-635.

35. Telfer, A. 2002. What is Beta-carotene Doing in the Photosystem II Reaction Centre? *Phil. Transact. Roy. Soc. B: Biol. Sci.* 357:1431-1470.

36. Dowling, J. E. 2000. George Wald. In *Biographical Memoirs National Academy of Sciences of the USA*. National Academic Press, Washington, DC. 299-317.

37. Dowling, J. E., and G. Wald. 1958. Vitamin A Deficiency and Night Blindness. *Proc. Natl. Acad. Sci. USA* 44:648-661.

38. Dowling, J. E., and G. Wald. 1960. The Biological Function of Vitamin A Acid. *Proc. Natl. Acad. Sci. USA* 46:587-608.

39. Clagett-Dame, M., and D. Knutson. 2011. Vitamin A in Reproduction and Development. *Nutrients* 3:385-428.

40. Wolbach, S. B., and P. R. Howe. 1925. Tissue Changes Following Deprivation of Fat-soluble A Vitamin. *J. Exp. Med.* 42:753-777.

41. Wolbach, S. B. 1937. The Pathologic Changes Resulting From Vitamin Deficiency. *J. Amer. Med. Soc.* 108:7-13.

42. Giguere, V., E. S. Ong, P. Segui, and R. M. Evans. 1987. Identification of a Receptor for the Morphogen Retinoic Acid. *Nature* 330:624-629.

43. Petkovich, M., N. J. Brand, A. Krust, and P. Chambon. 1987. A Human Retinoic Acid Receptor which Belongs to the Family of Nuclear Receptors. *Nature* 330:444-450.

44. Chambon, P. 1996. A Decade of Molecular Biology of Retinoic Acid Receptors. *Faseb J.* 10:940-954.

45. le Maire, A., and W. Bourguet. 2014. Retinoic Acid Receptors: Structural Basis for Coregulator Interaction and Exchange. *Sub-cellular Biochemistry* 70:37-54.

46. Balmer, J. E., and R. Blomhoff. 2002. Gene Expression Regulation by Retinoic Acid. *J. Lipid Res.* 43:1773-1808.

47. Smith, S. M., N. S. Levy, and C. E. Hayes. 1987. Impaired Immunity in Vitamin A-deficient Mice. *J. Nutr.* 117:857-865.

48. Pino-Lagos, K., Y. Guo, and R. J. Noelle. 2010. Retinoic Acid: A Key Player in Immunity. *BioFactors* 36:10.1002/biof.117.

49. Mora, J. R., M. Iwata, and U. H. von Andrian. 2008. Vitamin Effects on the Immune System: Vitamins A and D Take Centre Stage. *Nature Reviews. Immunology* 8:685-698.

50. Liu, Z. M., K. P. Wang, J. Ma, and S. Guo Zheng. 2015. The Role of All-trans Retinoic Acid in the Biology of Foxp3+ Regulatory T cells. *Cell. Mol. Immunol.* 12:553-557.

51. McGrane, M. M. 2007. Vitamin A Regulation of Gene Expression: Molecular Mechanism of a Prototype Gene. *The Journal of Nutritional Biochemistry* 18:497-508.

52. Savory, J. G. A., C. Edey, B. Hess, A. J. Mears, and D. Lohnes. 2014. Identification of Novel Retinoic Acid Target Genes. *Developmental Biology* 395:199-208.

53. Turfkruyer, M., A. Rekima, P. Macchiaverni, L. Le Bourhis, V. Muncan, G. R. van den Brink, M. K. Tulic, *et al.* 2015. Oral Tolerance

is Inefficient in Neonatal Mice Due to a Physiological Vitamin A Deficiency. *Mucosal Immunology* 9:479-491.

54. Moore, T., and P. D. Holmes. 1971. The Production of Experimental Vitamin A Deficiency in Rats and Mice. *Laboratory Animals* 5:239-250.

55. Trasino, S. E., Y. D. Benoit, and L. J. Gudas. 2015. Vitamin A Deficiency Causes Hyperglycemia and Loss of Pancreatic Beta-cell Mass. *J. Biol. Chem.* 290:1456-1473.

56. Wilson, J. G., C. B. Roth, and J. Warkany. 1953. An Analysis of the Syndrome of Malformations Induced by Maternal Vitamin A Deficiency. Effects of Restoration of Vitamin A at Various Times During Gestation. *The American Journal of Anatomy* 92:189-217.

57. Paiva, S. A., and R. M. Russell. 1999. Beta-carotene and Other Carotenoids as Antioxidants. *J. Am. Coll. Nutr.* 18:426-433.

58. Li, H., O. A. Sineshchekov, G. F. da Silva, and J. L. Spudich. 2015. In Vitro Demonstration of Dual Light-driven Na(+)/H(+) Pumping by a Microbial Rhodopsin. *Biophys. J.* 109:1446-1453.

59. Spudich, J. L., C. S. Yang, K. H. Jung, and E. N. Spudich. 2000. Retinylidene Proteins: Structures and Functions from Archaea to Humans. *Annual Review of Cell and Developmental Biology* 16:365-392.

60. Evidence for the convergent evolution of opsin proteins is summarized at http://evolutionarynovelty.blogspot.ca/2008/12/opsins-amazing- evolutionary-convergence.html.

61. Hammerling, U. 2013. The Centennial of Vitamin A: A Century of Research in Retinoids and Carotenoids. *Faseb J.* 27:3887-3890.

62. Semba, R. D. 2012. On the "Discovery" of Vitamin A. *Annals of Nutrition & Metabolism* 61:192-198.

63. Bloch, C. E. 1921. Clinical Investigation of Xerophthalmia and Dystrophy in Infants and Young Children. *J. Hygiene* 19:283-303.

64. Mori, M. 1904. Über den sogenante Hikan (Xerosis conjunctivae infantum ev. Keratomalacie). *Jahrbuch Kinderhelik* 59:175-195.

65. Blegvad, O. 1924. Xerophthalmia, Keratomalacia and Xerosis Conjunctivae. *Amer. J. Ophthalmology* 7:89-117.

---

66. Mellanby, E. 1926. A British Medical Association Journal Lecture on Diet and Disease. With Special Reference to the Teeth, Lungs, and Pre-Natal Feeding. *Brit. Med. J.* 1:515-519.
67. Green, H. N., and E. Mellanby. 1928. Vitamin A as an Anti-Infective Agent. *Brit. Med. J.* 2:691-696.
68. Green, H. N., D. Pindar, G. Davis, and E. Mellanby. 1931. Diet as a Prophylactic Agent Against Puerperal Sepsis. *Brit. Med. J.* 2:595-598.
69. Mori, S. 1922. The Changes in Para-ocular Glands which Follow the Administration of Diets Low in Fat-soluble A; with Notes of the Effects of the Same Diet on the Salivary Glands and Mucosa of the Larynx and Trachea. *Bull. Johns Hopkins Hospital* 33.
70. Ellison, J. B. 1932. Intensive Vitamin Therapy in Measles. *Brit. Med. J.* :708-711.
71. Scrimshaw, N. S., C. E. Taylor, and J. E. Gordon. 1968. *Interactions of Nutrition and Infection.* World Health Organization, Geneva.
72. Price, C. 2015. *The Vitamin Complex: Our Obsessive Quest for Nutritional Perfection.* Oneworld Publications, London.
73. Sommer, A. 1983. Mortality Associated with Mild, Untreated Xerophthalmia. *Trans. Amer. Opthalmol. Soc.* 81:825-853.
74. Sommer, A., I. Tarwotjo, G. Hussaini, and D. Susanto. 1983. Increased Mortality in Children with Mild Vitamin A Deficiency. *The Lancet* 2:585-588.
75. Sommer, A., I. Tarwotjo, E. Djunaedi, K. P. West, Jr., A. A. Loeden, R. Tilden, and L. Mele. 1986. Impact of Vitamin A Supplementation on Childhood Mortality. A Randomised Controlled Community Trial. *The Lancet* 1:1169-1173.
76. West, K. P., R. P. Pokhrel, J. Katz, S. C. LeClerq, S. K. Khatry, S. R. Shrestha, E. K. Pradhan, *et al.* 1991. Efficacy of Vitamin A in Reducing Preschool Child Mortality in Nepal. *The Lancet* 338:67-71.
77. Pokhrel, R. P., S. K. Khatry, K. P. West, Jr., S. R. Shrestha, J. Katz, E. K. Pradhan, S. C. LeClerq, *et al.* 1994. Sustained Reduction in Child Mortality with Vitamin A in Nepal. *The Lancet* 343:1368-1369.

78. Ghana VAST Study Team. 1993. Vitamin A Supplementation in Northern Ghana: Effects on Clinic Attendance, Hospital Admissions, and Child Mortality. *The Lancet* 342:7-12.

79. Sommer, A., and K. P. West Jr. 1996. *Vitamin A Deficiency. Health, Survival, and Vision.* Oxford University Press, New York.

80. Semba, R. D. 2001. The Vitamin A and Mortality Paradigm: Past, Present, and Future. *Scand. J. Nutr.* 45:46-50.

81. Beaton, G. H., R. Martorell, K. J. Aronson, B. Edmonston, A. C. Ross, B. Harvey, and G. McCabe. 1993. Effectiveness of Vitamin A Supplementation in the Control of Young Child Morbidity and Mortality in Developing Countries. *Canadian International Development Agency, Nutrition Policy Discussion Paper 13.*

82. Fawzi, W. W., T. C. Chalmers, M. G. Herrera, and F. Mosteller. 1993. Vitamin A Supplementation and Child Mortality. A Meta-analysis. *J. Amer. Med. Soc.* 269:898-903.

83. Mayo-Wilson, E., A. Imdad, K. Herzer, M. Y. Yakoob, and Z. A. Bhutta. 2011. Vitamin A Supplements for Preventing Mortality, Illness, and Blindness in Children Aged Under 5: Systematic Review and Meta-analysis. *Brit. Med. J.* 343:d5094.

84. West, K. P., Jr., J. Katz, S. K. Khatry, S. C. LeClerq, E. K. Pradhan, S. R. Shrestha, P. B. Connor, *et al.* 1999. Double Blind, Cluster Randomised Trial of Low Dose Supplementation with Vitamin A or Beta Carotene on Mortality Related to Pregnancy in Nepal. The NNIPS-2 Study Group. *Brit. Med. J.* 318:570-575.

85. Rice, A. L., K. P. J. West, and R. E. Black. 2004. Vitamin A Deficiency. In *Comparative Quantification of Health Risks. Global and Regional Burden of Disease Attributable to Selected Major Risk Factors.* A. D. L. M. Ezzati, A. Rodgers, and C. J. L. Murray, ed. World Health Organization, Geneva. 211-256.

86. Sommer, A. 2008. Vitamin A Deficiency and Clinical Disease: An Historical Overview. *J. Nutrition* 138:1835-1839.

87. Tang, G., Y. Hu, S. A. Yin, Y. Wang, G. E. Dallal, M. A. Grusak, and R. M. Russell. 2012. Beta-carotene in Golden Rice is as Good as

Beta-carotene in Oil at Providing Vitamin A to Children. *Amer. J. Clin. Nutr.* 96:658-664.

88. Gogia, S., and H. Sachdev. 2008. Vitamin A Supplementation for the Prevention of Morbidity and Mortality in Infants Six Months of Age or Less (Review). *Cochrane Database Systematic Review* CD007480.

89. WHO. 2013. *Micronutrient Deficiencies.* WHO, Geneva.

90. Bailey, R. L., K. P. West, Jr., and R. E. Black. 2015. The Epidemiology of Global Micronutrient Deficiencies. *Annals of Nutrition & Metabolism* 66 Suppl. 2:22-33.

91. Semba, R. D. 1999. Vitamin A and Immunity to Viral, Bacterial and Protozoan Infections. *Proc. Nutr. Soc.* 58:719-727.

92. Forrest, K. Y., and W. L. Stuhldreher. 2011. Prevalence and Correlates of Vitamin D Deficiency in US Adults. *Nutrition Research* 31:48-54.

93. Moertel, C. G., T. R. Fleming, E. T. Creagan, J. Rubin, M. J. O'Connell, and M. M. Ames. 1985. High-dose Vitamin C versus Placebo in the Treatment of Patients with Advanced Cancer Who have had No Prior Chemotherapy. A Randomized Double-blind Comparison. *N. Engl. J. Med.* 312:137-141.

94. Lipton, M. 1973. *Task Force Report on Megavitamin and Orthomolecular Therapy in Psychiatry.* American Psychiatric Association, Washington, DC.

95. Hemila, H., E. Chalker, and B. Douglas. 2007. Vitamin C for Preventing and Treating the Common Cold. *Cochrane Database of Systematic Reviews* 3:CD000980.

96. Mittal, M. K., T. Florin, J. Perrone, J. H. Delgado, and K. C. Osterhoudt. 2007. Toxicitiy from the Use of Niacin to Beat Urine Drug Screening. *Ann. Emergency Med.* 50:587-590.

97. Rodahl, K., and T. Moore. 1943. The Vitamin A Content and Toxicity of Bear and Seal Liver. *Biochem. J.* 37:166-168.

98. Penniston, K. L., and S. A. Tanumihardjo. 2006. The Acute and Chronic Toxic Effects of Vitamin A. *Amer. J. Clin. Nutr.* 83:191-201.

99. Dominguez, J., M. T. Hojyo, J. L. Celayo, L. Dominguez-Soto, and F. Teixeira. 1998. Topical Isotretinoin vs. Topical Retinoic Acid in the Treatment of Acne Vulgaris. *Int. J. Dermatol.* 37:54-55.

100. Walker, A., M. R. Zimmerman, and R. E. F. Leakey. 1982. A Possible Case of Hypervitaminosis A in Homo Erectus. *Nature* 296:248-250.

101. Rothman, K. J., L. L. Moore, M. R. Singer, U. S. Nguyen, S. Mannino, and A. Milunsky. 1995. Teratogenicity of High Vitamin A Intake. *N. Engl. J. Med.* 333:1369-1373.

102. Mills, J. L., J. L. Simpson, G. C. Cunningham, M. R. Conley, and G. G. Rhoads. 1997. Vitamin A and Birth Defects. *Amer. J. Obstet. Gynecol.* 177:31-36.

103. Rasmussen, K. 1998. *Safe Vitamin A Dosage During Pregnancy and Lactation. Recommendations and Report of a Consultation.* World Health Organization - The Micronutrient Initiative.

104. Wiegand, U. W., S. Hartmann, and H. Hummler. 1998. Safety of Vitamin A: Recent Results. *International Journal for Vitamin and Nutrition Research. Internationale Zeitschrift fur Vitamin- und Ernahrungsforschung. Journal international de vitaminologie et de nutrition* 68:411-416.

105. Bendich, A., and L. Langseth. 1989. Safety of Vitamin A. *Amer. J. Clin. Nutr.* 49:358-371.

106. Hummler, H., A. G. Hendrickx, and H. Nau. 1994. Maternal Toxicokinetics, Metabolism, and Embryo Exposure Following a Teratogenic Dosing Regimen with 13-cis-retinoic Acid (Isotretinoin) in the Cynomolgus Monkey. *Teratology* 50:184-193.

107. Ballard, M. S., M. Sun, and J. Ko. 2012. Vitamin A, Folate, and Choline as a Possible Preventive Intervention to Fetal Alcohol Syndrome. *Med. Hypoth.* 78:489-493.

108. Zachman, R. D., and M. A. Grummer. 1998. The Interaction of Ethanol and Vitamin A as a Potential Mechanism for the Pathogenesis of Fetal Alcohol Syndrome. *Alcoholism, Clinical and Experimental Research* 22:1544-1556.

109. Kot-Leibovich, H., and A. Fainsod. 2009. Ethanol Induces Embryonic Malformations by Competing for Retinaldehyde Dehydrogenase

Activity During Vertebrate Gastrulation. *Disease Models & Mechanisms* 2:295-305.

110. Young, J. K., H. E. Giesbrecht, M. N. Eskin, M. Aliani, and M. Suh. 2014. Nutrition Implications for Fetal Alcohol Spectrum Disorder. *Advances in Nutrition* 5:675-692.

111. Kumar, A., C. K. Singh, D. D. DiPette, and U. S. Singh. 2010. Ethanol Impairs Activation of Retinoic Acid Receptors in Cerebellar Granule Cells in a Rodent Model of Fetal Alcohol Spectrum Disorders. *Alcoholism, Clinical and Experimental Research* 34:928-937.

112. Johnson, C. S., R. M. Zucker, E. S. Hunter III, and K. K. Sulik. 2007. Perturbation of Retinoic Acid (RA)-mediated Limb Development Suggests a Role for Diminished RA Signaling in the Teratogenesis of Ethanol. *Birth Defects Research. Part A, Clinical and Molecular Teratology* 79:631-641.

113. Sempertegui, F., B. Estrella, V. Camaniero, V. Betancourt, R. Izurieta, W. Ortiz, E. Fiallo, *et al.* 1999. The Beneficial Effects of Weekly Low-dose Vitamin A Supplementation on Acute Lower Respiratory Infections and Diarrhea in Ecuadorian Children. *Pediatrics* 104:e1.

114. Carpenter, T. O., J. M. Pettifor, R. M. Russell, J. Pitha, S. Mobarhan, M. S. Ossip, S. Wainer, *et al.* 1987. Severe Hypervitaminosis A in Siblings: Evidence of Variable Tolerance to Retinol Intake. *J. Pediatrics* 111:507-512.

115. Florentino, R. F., C. C. Tanchoco, A. C. Ramos, T. S. Mendoza, E. P. Natividad, J. B. Tangco, and A. Sommer. 1990. Tolerance of Preschoolers to Two Dosage Strengths of Vitamin A Preparation. *Amer. J. Clin. Nutr.* 52:694-700.

116. West, K. P., R. D. W. Klemm, and A. Sommer. 2010. Vitamin A Saves Lives. Sound Science, Sound Policy. *J. World Public Health Nutrition Association* 1.

117. Wallace, S. K. 2012. Global Health in Conflict. Understanding Opposition to Vitamin A Supplementation in India. *Amer. J. Public Health* 102:1286-1297.

118. Mudur, G. 2001. Deaths Trigger Fresh Controversy over Vitamin A Programme in India. *Brit. Med. J.* 323:1206.

119. West, K. P., Jr., and A. Sommer. 2002. Vitamin A Programme in Assam Probably Caused Hysteria. *Brit. Med. J.* 324:791.

120. Michaelsson, K., H. Lithell, B. Vessby, and H. Melhus. 2003. Serum Retinol Levels and the Risk of Fracture. *N. Engl. J. Med.* 348:287-294.

121. Conaway, H. H., P. Henning, and U. H. Lerner. 2013. Vitamin A Metabolism, Action, and Role in Skeletal Homeostasis. *Endocrine Reviews* 34:766-797.

122. Tang, G., J. Qin, G. G. Dolnikowski, R. M. Russell, and M. A. Grusak. 2005. Spinach or Carrots can Supply Significant Amounts of Vitamin A as Assessed by Feeding with Intrinsically Deuterated Vegetables. *Amer. J. Clin. Nutr.* 82:821-828.

123. Ziegler, R. G., S. T. Mayne, and C. A. Swanson. 1996. Nutrition and Lung Cancer. *Cancer Causes Control* 7:157-177.

124. Omenn, G. S., G. E. Goodman, M. D. Thornquist, J. Balmes, M. R. Cullen, A. Glass, J. P. Keogh*, et al.* 1996. Effects of a Combination of Beta Carotene and Vitamin A on Lung Cancer and Cardiovascular Disease. *N. Engl. J. Med.* 334:1150-1155.

125. Neuhouser, M. L., R. E. Patterson, M. D. Thornquist, G. S. Omenn, I. B. King, and G. E. Goodman. 2003. Fruits and Vegetables are Associated with Lower Lung Cancer Risk Only in the Placebo Arm of the Beta-carotene and Retinol Efficacy Trial (CARET). *Cancer Epidemiol. Biomarkers Prev.* 12:350-358.

126. Sayin, V. I., M. X. Ibrahim, E. Larssons, J. A. Nilsson, P. Lindahl, and M. O. Bergo. 2014. Antioxidants Accelerate Lung Cancer Progression in Mice. *Sci. Transl. Med.* 6:221ra215.

127. Le Gal, K., M. X. Ibrahim, C. Wiel, V. I. Sayin, M. K. Akula, C. Karlsson, M. G. Dalin*, et al.* 2015. Antioxidants can Increase Melanoma Metastasis in Mice. *Sci. Transl. Med.* 7:308re308.

128. Pirie, A. 1977. Effects of Locally Applied Retinoic Acid on Corneal Xerophthalmia in the Rat. *Experimental Eye Research* 25:297-302.

129. Sommer, A. 1983. Treatment of Corneal Xerophthalmia with Topical Retinoic Acid. *Am. J. Ophthalmol.* 95:349-352.

130. Weiss, J. S., C. N. Ellis, J. T. Headington, T. Tincoff, T. A. Hamilton, and J. J. Voorhees. 1988. Topical Tretinoin Improves Photoaged

Skin. A Double-blind Vehicle-controlled Study. *J. Amer. Med. Soc.* 259:527-532.

131. Cho, S., L. Lowe, T. A. Hamilton, G. J. Fisher, J. J. Voorhees, and S. Kang. 2005. Long-term Treatment of Photoaged Human Skin with Topical Retinoic Acid Improves Epidermal Cell Atypia and Thickens the Collagen Band in Papillary Dermis. *J. Amer. Acad. Dermatol.* 53:769-774.

132. Sorg, O., and J. H. Saurat. 2014. Topical Retinoids in Skin Ageing: A Focused Update with Reference to Sun-induced Epidermal Vitamin A Deficiency. *Dermatology* 228:314-325.

133. Ministry of Health and National Institute of Public Health. 2001. *Report on National Health Survey: Health Status of the People in Lao PDR*. Ventiane, Lao PDR.

134. Ahmed, F. 1999. Vitamin A Deficiency in Bangladesh: A Review and Recommendations for Improvement. *Public Health Nutr.* 2:1-14.

135. UNICEF. 2015. *2014 Annual Results Report - Nutrition*. UNICEF, New York.

136. Gopalan, C. 2008. Vitamin A Deficiency—Overkill. *NFI Bulletin* 29:1-3.

137. Mason, J., T. Greiner, R. Shrimpton, D. Sanders, and J. Yukich. 2015. Vitamin A Policies Need Rethinking. *Int. J. Epidemiol.* 44:283-292.

138. Latham, M. 2010. The Great Vitamin A Fiasco. *World Nutrition* 1:12-45.

139. Ramakrishnan, U., M. C. Latham, R. Abel, and E. A. Frongillo. 1995. Vitamin A Supplementation and Morbidity among Preschool Children in South India. *Amer. J. Clin. Nutr.* 61:1295-1303.

140. Awasthi, S., R. Peto, S. Read, S. Clark, V. Pande, and D. Bundy. 2013. Vitamin A Supplementation Every 6 Months with Retinol in 1 Million Pre-school Children in North India: DEVTA, a Cluster-randomised Trial. *The Lancet* 381:1469-1477.

141. Sommer, A., K. P. West, Jr., and R. Martorell. 2013. Vitamin A Supplementation in Indian Children. *The Lancet* 382:591.

142. Mannar, K., W. Schultink, and K. Spahn. 2013. Vitamin A Supplementation in Indian Children. *The Lancet* 382:591-592.

143. Bhutia, D. T., S. de Pee, and P. A. C. Zwanikken. 2013. Vitamin A Coverage among Under-five Children. A Critical Appraisal of the Vitamin A Supplementation Program in India. *Sight and Life* 27:12-19.

144. Sommer, A. 1990. Xerophthalmia, Keratomalacia and Nutritional Blindness. *Int. Ophthalmol.* 14:195-199.

145. Arlappa, N. 2011. Vitamin A Deficiency is Still a Public Health Problem in India. *Indian Pediatrics* 48:853-854.

146. Zimmerman, M. B. 2008. Research on Iodine Deficiency and Goiter in the 19th and Early 20th Centuries. *J. Nutr.* 138:2060-2063.

147. Troen, A. M., B. Mitchell, B. Sorensen, M. H. Wener, A. Johnston, B. Wood, J. Selhub, *et al.* 2006. Unmetabolized Folic Acid in Plasma is Associated with Reduced Natural Killer Cell Cytotoxicity among Postmenopausal Women. *J. Nutr.* 136:189-194.

148. Smith, A. D., Y. I. Kim, and H. Refsum. 2008. Is Folic Acid Good for Everyone? *Amer. J. Clin. Nutr.* 87:517-533.

149. Dary, O., and J. O. Mora. 2002. Food Fortification to Reduce Vitamin A Deficiency: International Vitamin A Consultative Group Recommendations. *J. Nutr.* 132:2927s-2933s.

150. Arroyave, G., L. A. Mejia, and J. R. Aguilar. 1981. The Effect of Vitamin A Fortification of Sugar on the Serum Vitamin A Levels of Preschool Guatemalan Children: a Longitudinal Evaluation. *Amer. J. Clin. Nutr.* 34:41-49.

151. Dary, O., and J. O. Mora. 2002. Food Fortification to Reduce Vitamin A Deficiency: International Vitamin A Consultative Group Recommendations. *J. Nutr.* 132:2927S-2933S.

152. Haskell, M. J., K. M. Jamil, F. Hassan, J. M. Peerson, M. I. Hossain, G. J. Fuchs, and K. H. Brown. 2004. Daily Consumption of Indian Spinach (Basella Alba) or Sweet Potatoes has a Positive Effect on Total-body Vitamin A Stores in Bangladeshi Men. *Amer. J. Clin. Nutr.* 80:705-714.

153. Van Loo-Bouwman, C. A., T. H. Naber, and G. Schaafsma. 2014. A Review of Vitamin A Equivalency of Beta-carotene in Various Food Matrices for Human Consumption. *Br J. Nutr.* 111:2153-2166.

154. Muzhingi, T., T. H. Gadaga, A. H. Siwela, M. A. Grusak, R. M. Russell, and G. Tang. 2011. Yellow Maize with High Beta-carotene is an Effective Source of Vitamin A in Healthy Zimbabwean Men. *Amer. J. Clin. Nutr.* 94:510-519.

155. de Pee, S., C. E. West, Muhilal, D. Karyadi, and J. G. Hautvast. 1995. Lack of Improvement in Vitamin A Status with Increased Consumption of Dark-green Leafy Vegetables. *The Lancet* 346:75-81.

156. van Jaarsveld, P. J., M. Faber, S. A. Tanumihardjo, P. Nestel, C. J. Lombard, and A. J. S. Benadé. 2005. β-carotene-rich Orange-fleshed Sweet Potato Improves the Vitamin A Status of Primary School Children Assessed with the Modified-relative-dose-response Test. *Amer. J. Clin. Nutr.* 81:1080-1087.

157. HarvestPlus. 2010. *Reaching and Engaging End Users (REU) with Orange Fleshed Sweet Potato (OFSP) in East and Southern Africa. Final Report to the Bill and Melinda Gates Foundation.*

158. Low, J. W., M. Arimond, N. Osman, B. Cunguara, F. Zano, and D. Tschirley. 2007. A Food-based Approach Introducing Orange-fleshed Sweet Potatoes Increased Vitamin A Intake and Serum Retinol Concentrations in Young Children in Rural Mozambique. *J. Nutr.* 137:1320-1327.

159. Jones, K. M., and A. deBrauw. 2015. Using Agriculture to Improve Child Health: Promoting Orange Sweet Potatoes Reduces Diarrhea. *World Development* 74:15-24.

160. Hotz, C., C. Loechl, A. Lubowa, J. K. Tumwine, G. Ndeezi, A. Nandutu Masawi, R. Baingana, *et al.* 2012. Introduction of β-carotene-rich Orange Sweet Potato in Rural Uganda Results in Increased Vitamin A Intakes among Children and Women and Improved Vitamin A Status among Children. *J. Nutr.* 142:1871-1880.

161. Saltzman, A., E. Birol, H. E. Bouis, E. Boy, F. F. DeMoura, Y. Islam, and W. H. Pfeiffer. 2014. Biofortification: Progress Toward a More Nourishing Future. In *Bread and Brain, Education and Poverty*. Pontifical Academy of Sciences, Vatican City. 1-23.

162. Lamberts, L., and J. A. Delcour. 2008. Carotenoids in Raw and Parboiled Brown and Milled Rice. *J. Agric. Food Chem.* 56:11914-11919.

163. Bevan, M. W., R. B. Flavell, and M.-D. Chilton. 1983. A Chimaeric Antibiotic Resistance Gene as a Selectable Marker for Plant Cell Transformation. *Nature* 304:184-187.

164. Herrera-Estrella, L., A. Depicker, M. Van Montagu, and J. Schell. 1983. Expression of Chimaeric Genes Transferred into Plant Cells Using a Ti-plasmid-derived Vector. *Nature* 303:209-213.

165. Fraley, R. T., S. G. Rogers, R. B. Horsch, P. R. Sanders, J. S. Flick, S. P. Adams, M. L. Bittner, *et al.* 1983. Expression of Bacterial Genes in Plant Cells. *Proc. Natl. Acad. Sci. USA* 80:4803-4807.

166. Kyndt, T., D. Quispe, H. Zhai, R. Jarret, M. Ghislain, Q. Liu, G. Gheysen, *et al.* 2015. The Genome of Cultivated Sweet Potato Contains Agrobacterium T-DNAs with Expressed Genes: An Example of a Naturally Transgenic Food Crop. *Proc. Natl. Acad. Sci. USA* 112:5844-5849.

167. Ye, X., S. Al-Babili, A. Kloti, J. Zhang, P. Lucca, P. Beyer, and I. Potrykus. 2000. Engineering the Provitamin A (Beta-carotene) Biosynthetic Pathway into (Carotenoid-free) Rice Endosperm. *Science* 287:303-305.

168. Paine, J. A., C. A. Shipton, S. Chaggar, R. M. Howells, M. J. Kennedy, G. Vernon, S. Y. Wright, *et al.* 2005. Improving the Nutritional Value of Golden Rice through Increased Pro-vitamin A Content. *Nature Biotechnol.* 23:482-487.

169. Enserink, M. 2008. Tough Lessons From Golden Rice. *Science* 320:468-471.

170. Dubock, A. 2014. The Present Status of Golden Rice. *J. Huazhong Agricultural University* 33. :69-84

171. Tang, G., J. Qin, G. G. Dolnikowski, R. M. Russell, and M. A. Grusak. 2009. Golden Rice is an Effective Source of Vitamin A. *Amer. J. Clin. Nutr.* 89:1776-1783.

172. Dubock, A. 2014. The Politics of Golden Rice. *GM Crops & Food* 5:210-222.

173. The press conference describing this situation can be found at http://www.goldenrice.org/PDFs/China_nutr_rep_2004_en.pdf.

174. Alberts, B., R. Beachy, D. Baulcombe, G. Blobel, S. Datta, N. Fe-doroff, D. Kennedy, *et al.* 2013. Standing Up for GMOs. *Science* 341:1320.

175. This statement can be found at http://www.democraciaycooperacion.net/espacio-colaborativo/asia-pacific/your-documents-attached-to-the/article/philippines-apc-hails-uprooting-of.

176. The court decision is given at http://www.ensser.org/fileadmin/files/NoticeOfDecision-CA-G.R.SP-No.00013.pdf. Dr. Malakyang's comments are on page 14 of the original document.

177. Pedro, M. R., J. R. Madriaga, C. V. Barba, R. C. Habito, A. E. Gana, M. Deitchler, and J. B. Mason. 2004. The National Vitamin A Supplementation Program and Subclinical Vitamin A Deficiency among Preschool Children in the Philippines. *Food and Nutrition Bulletin* 25:319-329.

178. Kapil, U., and H. P. S. Sachdev. 2013. Massive Dose Vitamin A Pro-gramme in India - Need for a Targeted Approach. *Indian J. Med. Res.* 138:411-417.

179. This number comes from the International Rice Research Institute in Manila, posted at http://irri.org/golden-rice/faqs/why-is-golden-rice-needed-in-the-philippines-since-vitamin-a-deficiency-is-already-decreasing.

180. Stevens, G. A., J. E. Bennett, Q. Hennocq, Y. Lu, L. M. De-Re-gil, L. Rogers, G. Danaei, *et al.* 2015. Trends and Mortality Effects of Vitamin A Deficiency in Children in 138 Low-income and Mid-dle-income Countries Between 1991 and 2013: A Pooled Analysis of Population-based Surveys. *The Lancet Global Health* 3:e528-536.

181. These figures were posted on the FNRI website at http://www1.fnri.dost.gov.ph/images/stories/8thNNS/fnri_facts%26figures2011.pdf.

182. Smith, T. W., and J. Son. 2013. *Trends in Public Attitudes About Confidence in Institutions.* General Social Survey 2012 Final Report. NORC, University of Chicago, Chicago, IL.

183. Taubes, G. 2001. Nutrition. The Soft Science of Dietary Fat. *Science* 291:2536-2545.

184. J., B. 2015. Many Psychology Papers Fail Replication Test. *Science* 349:910-911.

185. Prinz, F., T. Schlange, and K. Asadullah. 2011. Believe It or Not: How Much Can We Rely on Published Data on Potential Drug Targets? *Nature Rev. Drug Discovery* 10:712.

186. These numbers are summarized at http://www.pewinternet. org/2015/01/29/public-and-scientists-views-on-science-and-society/.

187. This report can be found at https://ec.europa.eu/research/biosociety/ pdf/a_decade_of_eu-funded_gmo_research.pdf.

188. Chokshi, N. 2016. Stop Bashing GMO Foods, More Than 100 Nobel Laureates Say. *New York Times,* June 30.

189. McWilliams, J. E. 2009. *Just Food.* Little, Brown and Co., New York.

190. Federoff, N., and N. M. Brown. 2004. *Mendel in the Kitchen.* Joseph Henry Press, Washington, DC.

191. Klümper, W., and M. Qaim. 2014. A Meta-analysis of the Impacts of Genetically Modified Crops. *PLos One* 9:e111629.

192. Aris, A., and S. Leblanc. 2011. Maternal and Fetal Exposure to Pesticides Associated to Genetically Modified Foods in Eastern Townships of Quebec, Canada. *Reprod. Toxicol.* 31:528-533.

193. Seralini, G. E., E. Clair, R. Mesnage, S. Gress, N. Defarge, M. Malatesta, D. Hennequin, *et al.* 2012. Long Term Toxicity of a Roundup Herbicide and a Roundup-tolerant Genetically Modified Maize. *Food and Chemical Toxicology : An International Journal Published for the British Industrial Biological Research Association* 50:4221-4231.

INDEX

ACKNOWLEDGEMENTS

I thank Alfred Sommer, Adrian Dubock, Jan Low, John Dowling, Zulfiqar Bhutta, and Bob Chow for information and advice on vitamin A-related subjects. I am grateful for the encouragement of Reinhard Illner, Sandy Briggs, Rod Edwards, Rod MacLeod, and Jennifer Kaufman-Shaw, and the editorial work of Dania Sheldon and design by Alex Hennig. The beginnings of this book can be traced to the Science Communication workshop held in Banff, Alberta, in the Spring of 2006.

www.ingramcontent.com/pod-product-compliance
Lightning Source LLC
Chambersburg PA
CBHW031931190326
41519CB00007B/487